T3-BEA-406

Instructor's Resource Manual and Testbank to Accompany

Essentials of
Nursing Research

METHODS, APPRAISAL, AND UTILIZATION

FIFTH EDITION

Denise F. Polit, PhD

President
Humanalysis, Inc.
Saratoga Springs, New York

Cheryl Tatano Beck, DNSc, CNM, FAAN

Professor
University of Connecticut, School of Nursing
Storrs, Connecticut

Bernadette P. Hungler, BSN, PhD

Visiting Lecturer
Regis College
Weston, Massachusetts

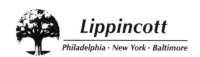

Lippincott

Philadelphia · New York · Baltimore

*Instructor's Resource Manual
and Testbank to Accompany*

Essentials of
Nursing Research

METHODS, APPRAISAL, AND UTILIZATION

FIFTH EDITION

Ancillary Editor: *Doris S. Wray*
Compositor: *Pine Tree Composition*
Prnter/Binder: *R.R. Donnelly*

Copyright © 2001 by Lippincott Williams & Wilkins. All rights reserved. No part of this book may be used or reproduced in any manner whatsoever without written permission with the following exception: Testing materials may be copied for classroom use, provided the instructor has adopted its accompanying text, *Essentials of Nursing Research: Methods, Appraisal, and Utilization* by Denise F. Polit, Cheryl Tatano Beck, and Bernadette P. Hungler. Printed in the United States of America. For information write Lippincott Williams & Wilkins, 530 Walnut Street, Philadelphia, Pennsylvania 19106-3780.

ISBN: 0–7817–2559–3

Any procedure or practice described in this book should be applied by the health care practitioner under appropriate supervision in accordance with professional standards of care used with regard to the unique circumstances that apply in each practice situation. Care has been taken to confirm the accuracy of information presented and to describe generally accepted practices. However, the authors, editors, and publisher cannot accept any responsibility for errors or omissions or for any consequences from application of the information in this book and make no warranty, express or implied, with respect to the contents of the book.

Preface

■ Overview

Learning about the techniques of scientific research can be a boring and anxiety-provoking enterprise for students. There is new jargon to learn and tedious details to memorize in research textbooks. And many research reports—especially those describing quantitative studies—include dense tables and intimidating-looking symbols and are written in an uninviting, impersonal style. In preparing this textbook, we have tried to balance rigorous and factual content with a presentation designed to minimize fears, generate enthusiasm for the research process, and offer concrete support in students' efforts to evaluate and utilize research findings.

We recognize, however, that our role in accomplishing this objective is small relative to your own. We hope that, with the textbook, the Study Guide, and this Instructor's Resource Manual, we are providing you with some basic tools for communicating what research is all about, what it can accomplish, and how it can be used. We believe that learning about research methods is analogous to learning how to play a musical instrument: It may be somewhat painful and tedious in the beginning, but acquiring the skills opens up the possibility of a lifetime of growth and professional reward.

The textbook has been written primarily for undergraduate students—that is, for students who are learning how to critically read and appraise research reports. In this edition, a conscious effort was made to write as clearly and simply as possible. The textbook covers the standard content of graduate-level research methods textbooks, but in less depth and with a clearer emphasis on the needs of research consumers. The length should be manageable in a one-semester course.

Each chapter of the textbook contains explicit guidelines to assist readers in reviewing and critiquing aspects of a research report. Additionally, each chapter concludes with a brief description of actual nursing research studies—typically, one quantitative and one qualitative study—that students are asked to evaluate with respect to the issues covered in the chapter. Students could be asked to read relevant portions of the actual research report, so that they could do a more thorough evaluation. The studies that we selected are generally recent, methodologically excellent examples with respect to the content of the chapter. The Instructor's Manual includes comments on these actual research examples to help you prepare for classroom discussions.

An important point to emphasize is that doing research involves numerous methodologic decisions that affect the validity and integrity of the study. Any research problem can be studied in any number of ways—and different decisions can affect the results. Students need to become aware that simply because a report has been published does not mean that the researchers designed the best possible study. Thus, a major challenge to students is to consider improvements in study design and to recognize the implications of study limitations when interpreting study results. An equally compelling challenge is for students to envision using the results of research studies in their own clinical practice.

Another important lesson that students will hopefully grasp quickly is that research ideas don't just "happen," nor are they generated solely by researchers working in isolation from the real world. They are created out of curiosity about how the world functions and how human beings behave or experience things. Suggestions for research can be developed by *anyone*. Skills in research methods are essential to the conduct of a rigorous study, but not to its general conception. This point is particularly important for undergraduate students, who are bombarded with "facts" of clinical relevance without perhaps recognizing that, to get those "facts," people had to ask questions and seek answers to them. We hope that the textbook will help stimulate students to ask questions and to search for answers in the research literature—or in their own research.

■ Special Comments on Changes to the Fifth Edition

Much of the content of this fifth edition is similar to that in the previous edition of the textbook. Like the fourth edition, qualitative and quantitative research methods are given essentially the same degree of coverage. The textbook offers explicit comparisons between the two research approaches on all major issues, including problem selection, study design, sampling, data collection methods, and data analysis.

However, in this edition there is considerably more emphasis on reading and comprehending research reports and on research utilization. We have included a new chapter (Chapter 3) on how to read research reports. Tips on what to expect in research reports are interspersed throughout the chapters, rather than in separate sections at the end of each chapter. We believe that this approach will enhance the utility of these consumer tips, which are designed to help students make the transition between abstract principles of research methodology and specific features of studies reported in nursing journals.

With respect to utilization, we endeavored in this edition to tie chapter content to utilization throughout the book. For example, each research example at the end of each chapter now includes a discussion of the possible clinical relevance of the study. The final chapter on utilization has also been expanded and strengthened.

We are very enthusiastic about the revisions made in this edition. We hope the changes we have made will better meet the needs of students.

■ Some Comments on the Study Guide

We have indicated our purposes in creating an accompanying Study Guide in the preface to that volume. We have three additional comments to instructors using the workbook.

First, new to this edition is a CD-ROM with a testbank that students can use to review textbook material. There are generally ten to twenty multiple choice questions per chapter. The testbank has been designed to provide immediate feedback—information on why incorrect answers are wrong and why correct answers are right.

Second, as in the past, we do not recommend using the "Matching Exercises" and "Completion Exercises" as test questions. They were not developed with this purpose in mind. Indeed, many of the items could rightfully be challenged as "trick questions" if they were used in a testing situation. We view them as heuristic devices—as aids to help students review and apply material covered in the textbook. Therefore, we recommend having students complete these exercises in an open-book fashion.

Finally, we want to note that we have filled the Study Guide with hundreds of research possibilities to stimulate the students' imagination. It is our hope that, through the many examples in the textbook and the Study Guide, students will appreciate that research is undertaken because of curiosity and because of a desire to improve nursing care.

■ Some Comments on the Instructor's Resource Manual

Like the Study Guide, a chapter in this manual corresponds to each chapter in the textbook. Each chapter of the manual contains the following:

- *Statement of Intent.* Chapters are introduced with a discussion of the major purposes of the chapter, usually accompanied by our suggestions for which portions merit particular emphasis.
- *Comments on the Actual Research Examples in the Textbook.* High-quality studies were selected as actual research examples in the textbook. Therefore, most of the comments in this Instructor's Resource Manual

point out *why*, and in what way, the study is methodologically sound. However, methodologic concerns are also noted.

- *Answers to Selected Study Guide Exercises.* Answers to those questions that have reasonably objective "right" and "wrong" answers, such as the questions in the Matching and Completion Exercises are included. These answers also appear in the Appendix to the Study Guide. Additionally, the Instructor's Manual includes comments on the fictitious research examples in the Application Exercises.

- *Test Questions and Answers.* Multiple Choice and True/False test questions appear at the end of every chapter as well as provided in a generic electronic file format.

- *Transparency Masters.* Transparency Masters are easily designed to help prepare overheads for lectures, demonstration, and/or discussion.

We hope that this manual will help you and your students derive a maximally profitable experience from the textbook.

Contents

PART VI
Critical Appraisal and Utilization of Nursing Research

PART I

Overview of Nursing Research

CHAPTER 1

Exploring Nursing Research

■ Statement of Intent

A major purpose of this introductory chapter is to establish a foundation for understanding the role of disciplined research in the nursing profession. The chapter provides a brief history of nursing research and discusses the types of problem that nurse researchers have attempted to solve. A fundamental goal of the chapter is to show that research methods have relevance to the practice of nursing. We hope that students will come to appreciate that nursing research is not just for academics; it is for everyone who wants to solve problems or answer questions in a systematic way, and it is also for practicing nurses who must evaluate whether study results should be used as a basis for clinical practice. Chapter 1 discusses the many research-related roles that nurses might adopt along the consumer–producer continuum.

The chapter also presents an overview of the two paradigms (positivist and naturalistic) within which nursing studies are being conducted. It provides a basis for understanding the fundamental philosophical differences between the two paradigms and links the paradigms to methodologic strategies for acquiring knowledge. Throughout the textbook, distinctions between qualitative and quantitative research are noted, and so it is important for students to grasp the paradigmatic underpinnings of these approaches. The textbook adopts the view that both quantitative and qualitative research have important roles to play in nursing. However, both approaches have limitations, and these should also be understood by students.

■ Selected Comments on the Research Examples in the Textbook

RESEARCH EXAMPLE OF A QUANTITATIVE STUDY

The study by Stevens and her colleagues (1999) is a good example of a scientific study undertaken by a team of nurse researchers. Here are a few comments relating to the overall study:

- The study clearly has clinical relevance. However, replications of the study are needed, as well as further research on long-term effects.
- The study falls within a research priority area designated within CORP#1, namely research on low birthweight infants.

- The study used a traditional scientific approach within the positivist paradigm. Empirical evidence (i.e., measures of pain and heart rate) was collected in a systematic fashion from a reasonably large sample of children.

- Appropriately, the study was quantitative. The researchers obtained measures of several pain variables and of heart rate. Pain can be examined qualitatively, but heart rate cannot. In this example, the investigators were interested in documenting, in quantitative terms, the degree to which pain was affected by a specific intervention.

- The study has explanation as an implicit goal; that is, the researchers are really interested in answering the question: What factors affect (reduce) pain in low birthweight? The more direct purposes of the investigation, however, are prediction and control. The researchers, as a result of their study, can tentatively predict that giving infants pacifiers with sucrose will reduce pain (while infant position will not), and they therefore can exert some control over pain.

- The study's aim is applied in nature: The researchers were testing the efficacy of specific nursing interventions.

RESEARCH EXAMPLE OF A QUALITATIVE STUDY

The study by Nehls (1999) is a good example of a qualitative study designed to provide important information on health issues. Here are a few comments relating to the overall study.

- The study is clearly relevant to the practice of nursing. It focuses on health issues for a group that has received inadequate research attention in the past.

- The naturalistic paradigm, appropriately, provides the underpinnings for this research. The researchers realized that the meaning of being diagnosed with borderline personality is complex and poorly understood. To gain insights into the phenomenon, it was essential to talk to patients with borderline personality directly and to probe deeply into the meanings and practices of this group. It was important for the researcher to understand how these women experienced their psychiatric illness, without imposing any controls or constraints on the research situation.

- The women's perceptions, emotions, and experiences in living with a diagnosis of borderline personality would have been difficult to measure quantitatively. In-depth, qualitative information had the greatest potential to offer insights.

- Like many qualitative studies, this study can be described as exploratory. When a new area is being researched, an exploratory study can provide insights on the full nature and meaning of the phenomenon of interest. An exploratory study can lay the groundwork for more focused research.

■ Answers to Selected Study-Guide Exercises

A.1.   1. a   2. b   3. c   4. c   5. b   6. a   7. c   8. a   9. c   10. d

A.2.   1. a   2. b   3. d   4. a   5. b   6. a   7. b   8. d   9. b   10. c
       11. a   12. a

B.1. Florence Nightingale 2. Nursing education   3. Clinical practice
   4. Tradition   5. Inductive   6. Logical positivism
                                                       (positivism)
   7. Determinism   8. Naturalistic   9. Scientific approach
  10. Empirical   11. Generalization   12. Reductionist
  13. Field   14. Quantitative research 15. Qualitative re-
                                                       search
  16. Identification

C.5.   a. Basic   b. Applied   c. Applied   d. Basic   e. Basic
         f. Applied g. Basic   h. Applied

D.2.   Nicolet's study has direct clinical relevance to the practice of nursing. The study is designed to provide information that could be used by other nurses to promote the health and well-being of a vulnerable group, the elderly.

The study adheres to the classical scientific approach within a positivism tradition. Nicolet was attempting to gain systematic knowledge about the effect of alternative techniques of persuasion on the behavior of high-risk elderly citizens through direct empirical observation. She controlled the situation by sending half the members of the senior citizens' center a positively worded message (i.e., stressing the health benefits of a flu shot) and the other half a negatively worded message (i.e., stressing the health risks of failure to get a flu shot). The behavior of interest, whether the person comes forward for a flu shot, will be directly observable by the researcher. Because the alternative letters were mailed to the elderly impartially (i.e., an elderly person was equally likely to be sent a negatively worded as a positively worded letter) and because the letters were similar in other respects (e.g., both groups were advised of the free transportation and immunizations), we can conclude that the research was characterized by a fairly high degree of control. Although Nicolet was observing the behavioral responses of 500 specific elderly citizens, she is presumably interested in generalizing the results more broadly so that others can adopt the most effective strategy for encouraging preventive health practices among the elderly.

Nicolet's study, as described here, appears not to have an explanatory purpose. At the end of the research, she may learn that one type of communication approach is better than the other, but she will not know *why*. Perhaps, then, this study should be characterized as exploratory, but it can also serve a predictive and control function (e.g., health care workers can, in the future, predict that a certain approach is more likely to yield high rates of compliance and may want to control subsequent campaigns accordingly).

Nicolet's research is applied in nature. She presumably wanted information that would be helpful in developing communication strategies or health care policies for the elderly. This is essentially a utilitarian function.

The basic research question concerns *how many* of the elderly in the two groups come forward to receive a flu shot, and therefore quantitative information was needed. The difference in rates of coming forward would be analyzed using quantitative (statistical) procedures. It is important to note, however, that the study might well be enhanced through the collection of some qualitative information as well. For example, the researcher could contact noncompliers from both groups to ask them if they understood the content of the letter and to seek their general reaction to the message. These people could also be asked why they did not come to the clinic for a flu shot. Thus, even studies that have a positivist framework can sometimes be enhanced by questions that are associated with a naturalistic perspective.

D.3.   Ryan's study delved into an intensely personal and complex area of human experience, an area that has not yet been carefully researched. Individuals who have lost a parent to a genetically linked disease must develop effective strategies for assessing and managing risk. Health care professionals can perhaps facilitate risk management if they better understand the risk experience from the perspective of those who are experiencing it. Thus, Ryan's study has the potential to be clinically significant.

The nature of the research problem is well-suited to an in-depth examination of the risk experience *as it is lived*—not as it is perceived or appraised by others. What the researcher wanted to study was the people's own interpretations of their experiences, and Ryan sought to obtain this knowledge by letting the individuals speak at length in their own words. By taping the interviews, the researcher was able to capture those words without having to take detailed notes, which can slow down and constrain the interview flow. Given the probing nature of the inquiry, the collection of narrative, subjective information was appropriate.

As suggested by the summary of the study, the researcher's purpose was both descriptive (what are the dimensions of the risk experience?) and exploratory (what is the full nature of the risk experience?). The study appears to be seeking knowledge primarily for knowledge's own sake (i.e., has a basic orientation), but it is not difficult to envision the uses to which that knowledge could be placed.

▪ Test Questions and Answers

MULTIPLE CHOICE

1. Which of the following groups would be *best* served by the development of a scientific base for nursing practice?
   a. Nursing administrators
   b. Nursing educators
   c. Practicing nurses
   *d. Nursing's clientele

2. An especially important goal for the nursing profession is to:
    a. Conduct research to better understand supply and demand for nurses
    *b. Establish a scientific base of knowledge for the improvement of practice
    c. Document the role nursing serves in society
    d. Establish research priorities

3. Which of the following is *not* a current priority for clinical nursing research?
    a. Cost-effective health care delivery systems
    b. Health promotion
    *c. Nurses' personalities
    d. Prevention of illness

4. Most nursing studies at mid-century focused on:
    a. Consumer satisfaction
    b. Clinical problems
    c. Health promotion
    *d. Nursing education

5. Which of the following topics most closely conforms to the priorities that have been suggested for future nursing research?
    a. Attitudes of nursing students toward smoking
    *b. Factors associated with patient compliance with treatment
    c. Nursing staff morale and turnover
    d. Number of doctorally prepared nurses in various clinical specialties

6. Deductive reasoning is the process of:
    a. Verifying assumptions that are part of our heritage
    *b. Developing specific predictions from general principles
    c. Empirically testing observations that are made known through our sense organs
    d. Forming generalizations from specific observations

7. To those espousing a naturalistic paradigm, there is an assumption that:
    a. A fixed reality exists in nature for humans to understand
    b. The nature of reality has changed over time
    *c. Reality is multiply constructed and multiply interpreted by humans
    d. Reality cannot be studied empirically

8. To those espousing a positivist paradigm, there is an assumption that:
    *a. The researcher is objective and independent of those being studied
    b. The researcher cannot interact with those being studied
    c. The researcher instructs those being studied to be objective in providing information
    d. The distance between the researcher and those being researched is minimized to enhance the interactive process

9. The traditional scientific approach is *not* characterized by which of the following attributes?
   a. Control over external factors
   b. Systematic measurement and observation of natural phenomena
   c. Logical reasoning
   *d. Emphasis on a holistic view of a phenomenon, studied in a rich context

10. Empiricism refers to:
   a. Making generalizations from specific observations
   b. Deducing specific predictions from generalizations
   *c. Gathering evidence rooted in objective reality
   d. Verifying the assumptions on which a study was based

11. A hallmark of the scientific approach is that it is:
   a. Infallible
   b. Holistic
   *c. Systematic
   d. Flexible

12. Which of the following limits the power of the scientific approach to answer questions about human life?
   a. The necessity of departing from traditional beliefs
   *b. The difficulty of measuring psychosocial characteristics of humans
   c. The inability to control potential biases
   d. The shortage of theories about human behavior

13. The scientific approach has its intellectual roots in:
   *a. Logical positivism
   b. Determinism
   c. Phenomenology
   d. Inductive reasoning

14. One of the criticisms of the scientific approach is that it is overly:
   a. Logical
   b. Deterministic
   c. Empirical
   *d. Reductionist

15. Naturalistic qualitative research typically
   a. Involves deductive processes
   b. Attempts to control the research context to better understand the nature of the phenomenon being studied
   *c. Takes place in the field
   d. Focuses on the idiosyncrasies of those being studied

16. Quantitative and qualitative research do *not* share which of the following features in common?
   a. A desire to gain an understanding of the true state of human affairs
   *b. Roots in nineteenth-century phenomenological thought
   c. Reliance on external evidence collected through the senses
   d. Utility to the nursing profession

17. A descriptive question that a qualitative researcher might ask is:
    - *a. What are the dimensions this phenomenon?
    - b. How frequently does this phenomenon occur?
    - c. What is the average duration of of this phenomenon?
    - d. How prevalent is this phenomenon?

18. A researcher wants to investigate the effect of patients' body position on blood pressure. The study would most likely be:
    - a. Qualitative
    - *b. Quantitative
    - c. Inductive
    - d. Insufficient information to determine

19. A researcher wants to study the process by which people make decisions about seeking treatment for infertility. The researcher's paradigmatic orientation most likely is:
    - a. Positivism
    - b. Determinism
    - c. Empiricism
    - *d. Naturalism

20. A researcher is studying the effect of massage on the alleviation of pain in cancer patients. The study would be described as:
    - a. Descriptive
    - b. Exploratory
    - *c. Applied
    - d. Basic

TRUE/FALSE

(F) 1. Throughout the history of nursing research, most studies have focused on clinical problems.

(F) 2. The journal *Nursing Research* began publication during the early 1900s.

(T) 3. Most people would agree that nursing research began with Florence Nightingale.

(F) 4. The federal agency that currently offers support for nursing research is the National Center for Nursing Research.

(F) 5. The current trend in nursing research is a focus on nursing administration.

(F) 6. The journal *Nursing Research* and two to three newer journals are currently the only journals for communicating the results of nursing research studies.

(T) 7. Journal clubs for practicing nurses involve meetings to discuss and critically evaluate research studies.

(F) 8. All producers of nursing research work in universities and schools of nursing.

(F) 9. Deductive reasoning is the process of developing generalizations from specific observations.

(T) 10. A paradigm is a general perspective on the nature of the real world.

(T) 11. According to the positivist paradigm, there is an objective reality that can be understood by researchers.

(F)   12. The naturalistic paradigm is associated with structured, quantitative research.

(T)   13. A naturalistic researcher attempts to understand rather than control the context of those being studied.

(F)   14. Nursing leaders currently are suggesting that in-depth, process-oriented studies are more important than controlled quantitative studies for nursing practice.

(F)   15. Empirical evidence is information derived from introspective analysis of real-world phenomena.

(T)   16. The scientific approach assumes that all phenomena have antecedent causes.

(T)   17. Quantitative researchers are more likely than qualitative researchers to pursue research with prediction and control as a purpose.

(F)   18. Quantitative researchers tend to emphasize the dynamic and holistic aspects of human experience.

(T)   19. Applied research is designed to solve immediate problems.

(F)   20. Research questions that focus on identification (e.g., What is this phenomenon?) are most likely to be applied in nature.

Comprehending the Research Process

■ Statement of Intent

The purpose of Chapter 2 is to provide students with some basic groundwork for dealing with the remainder of the text. There are two main parts to this chapter. The first part introduces research terminology that recurs throughout the text. The students' firm grounding in basic research terms should facilitate their ability to grasp more complex methodologic concepts later in the book and to begin to read research reports. This edition also distinguishes the basic terminology used by qualitative and quantitative researchers—for example, *subject* versus *informant*. A chart summarizing differences in terminology has been included.

The second part of the chapter provides an overview of the steps that a researcher undertakes in conducting a study. Separate sections are devoted to describing the general progression of activities in qualitative and quantitative studies.

■ Selected Comments on the Research Examples in the Textbook

RESEARCH EXAMPLE OF A QUANTITATIVE STUDY

The textbook provided a brief abstract of some aspects of a study by McCurren, Dowe, Rattle, and Looney (1999). The study examined the relationship between participation in a special intervention for depressed nursing home residents and changes in the residents' level of depression. Here are a few comments about that study, with specific reference to the concepts discussed in Chapter 2.

- As in most research reports, McCurren et al. did not explicitly label the independent and dependent variables. In this study, participation versus nonparticipation in the low-cost intervention strategy was the independent variable. Change in scores on the Geriatric Depression Scale (GDS) was the dependent variable.

- The independent variable (participation in the intervention) was a dichotomous categorical variable. Technically, the GDS score was a discrete variable with a large number of values (30), although the large range of possible scores makes it look like a continuous variable.

- Operational definitions of the variables were fully elaborated in the report. Detailed information was provided about how and when the variables were measured.

- The relationship between declines in depression and participation in the special intervention is presumably causal: The intervention caused the nursing home residents to have improved mental health.

- The investigators chose to conduct a quantitative study to enable them to test a specific hypothesis about the relationship between their variables using appropriate statistical procedures. Depression can be studied qualitatively, but not *measured* in such a way that declines could be systematically documented.

RESEARCH EXAMPLE OF A QUALITATIVE STUDY

A brief overview of an interesting study by Schaefer, Ladd, Lammers, and Echenberg (1999) was included in the textbook. A few comments on aspects of this study discussed in Chapter 2 follow:

- The phenomenon under study was a complex and multifaceted—the experience of living with ovarian cancer during the childbearing years. This phenomenon would have been difficult to fully understand using tightly structured quantitative methods. Moreover, because so little prior work had focused on the day-to-day experiences of ovarian cancer victims, a qualitative study was appropriate. The researchers did not know in advance what the experiences would be like. They allowed the key themes to emerge during the course of the interviews. Only after analyzing their data did Schaefer and her colleagues discover the major thirteen themes that characterized the women's experiences.

- There were no concepts in this study that could be described as "independent" or "dependent" variables. Nor, as is appropriate for qualitative studies, were there operational definitions of any variables.

- Given the researchers' interest in describing an ongoing experience, it was appropriate to collect data from their study participants on several occasions over an extended period. This allowed changes in their experience to occur.

- In describing the thirteen main themes in their report, the researchers included examples of *raw data*—that is, excerpts from interviews that exemplified the themes that emerged.

■ Answers to Selected Study Guide Exercises

A.1.   1.a   2.c   3.b   4.a   5.b   6.a   7.c   8.c

A.2.   1.a   2.b   3.c   4.b   5.a   6.a

      7.b   8.c   9.a   10.b   11.a   12.b

A.3.   1.b   2.c   3.b   4.a   5.c   6.c   7.c   8.c

B.1. Researcher, investigator
2. Subjects, study participants
3. Concepts
4. Variable
5. Categorical
6. Continuous
7. Independent variable
8. Dependent
9. Independent
10. Data
11. Operational definitions
12. Qualitative
13. Patterns of association
14. Cause-and-effect
15. Functional (associative)
16. Qualitative, quantitative
17. Quantitative
18. Research design
19. Sample
20. Empirical (data collection)
21. Data analysis
22. Pilot study
23. Research report
24. Dissemination
25. Gaining entrée
26. Saturation

D.2.   In Portnoy and Stamm's fictitious study, the nature of the patient's home environment was the independent variable, reaction to hospital noise was the dependent variable, and three additional (extraneous) variables are identified. The researchers' operational definitions are fairly well detailed but could be improved. For three of the variables (home environment, age, and gender), it would be possible for anyone to replicate the measurements according to the definitions given. For the remaining two variables, further specification is needed. For the dependent variable (reaction to hospital noise), we do not know whether scores ranged from 0 to 5—that is, the sum of responses to the five questions—or whether there was some other scoring procedure. We also do not know the basis for dividing subjects into satisfied or dissatisfied groups. The social class variable is also vaguely described. Does the intake form record *actual* employment (e.g., teacher, mechanic) or classes of employment (e.g., professional, managerial, technical)? How was this information translated into social class?

More important, Portnoy and Stamm's definitions were probably not as well conceptualized as possible. For example, for the independent variable (type of home environment), it might be advisable to add dimensions other than quantity of household members. Examples include the presence versus absence of children under 10 years of age, proportion of minors to adults in the household, number of televisions and radios in the household, and urban versus rural residence.

The dependent variable, too, could probably have been defined better or defined in alternative ways. One of the problems with the present definition is that it depends on subjects' recall at discharge rather than on patients' immediate reactions to noises. In addition to obtaining self-reports during hospitalization, the researchers could have had nurses record the number of patient complaints about noise levels.

One can imagine a causal *pathway* between the independent and dependent variables: The number of household members might affect people's tolerance for different noise levels, and hence their satisfaction with hospital noises. However, it cannot really be said that number of household members *causes* dissatisfaction with noise levels. In fact, it cannot even be assumed that number of household members *influences* the patient's reaction to noise. It might be that people who are generally more comfortable in an environment with a lot of activity and noise seek to establish larger households (e.g., they might have more children). In other words, there are a number of possible explanations for a relationship between household size and noise tolerance. The relationship would best be characterized as functional.

Aspects with the home environment and people's reactions to noise cannot be quantified, and hence a quantitative study is not inappropriate. However, we can also envision that an in-depth, qualitative look at the home environments of patients with different hospital experiences could also be profitable—and might suggest to a quantitative researcher the aspects of the home environment that are especially likely to be related to tolerance for hospital noise.

D.4.   The general phenomenon that Godine and Nicholson focused on was patients' views about the meaning of noncompliance with a therapeutic regimen. There are no "independent" and "dependent" variables in this investigation. Godine and Nicholson were not interested in what caused or influenced the patients' viewpoints, nor on what the consequences of those viewpoints were. Rather, they wanted to obtain personalized, subjective accounts of what noncompliance meant in the lives of chronically ill people. Such a focus is appropriate for a qualitative inquiry.

The brief summary presented in the Study Guide does not discuss whether the researchers examined patterns of association. Godine and Nicholson would not have known in advance (nor do we know from the description) whether interesting patterns might emerge—indeed, the point of an exploratory qualitative study is to let the data speak for themselves. However, it is very well possible that interesting patterns would have been detected and explored by the researcher. For example, one can imagine that men and women might have different viewpoints about compliance; the *nature* of the chronic illness might also play a role in the meaning of noncompliance.

Given that the study focused on a rural population, the researchers' decision to recruit study participants through a health clinic was probably a reasonable one. However, it might have been advisable to conduct the in-depth interviews in the settings in which noncompliance typically occurs—that is, in the homes of the participants, rather than in the clinic itself.

■ Test Questions and Answers

MULTIPLE CHOICE

1. Which of the following terms is *not* typically used by quantitative researchers to refer to people who participate in a study?
   *a. Informants
   b. Respondents
   c. Study participants
   d. Subjects

2. Which of the following terms is used by both qualitative and quantitative researchers to refer to the abstractions under study?
   *a. Concept
   b. Construct
   c. Phenomenon
   d. Variable

3. "Male" is:
   *a. Not a variable
   b. A categorical variable
   c. An independent variable
   d. A continuous variable

4. Of the following, the best example of a continuous variable is:
   a. Shift assignment
   b. Method of teaching
   *c. Blood pressure
   d. Blood type

5. "Pulse rate" is:
   a. Not a variable
   b. A categorical variable
   c. Inherently an independent variable
   *d. None of the above

6. "Nursing effectiveness" is:
   a. A concept
   b. A construct
   c. A variable
   *d. All of the above

7. The dependent variable(s) in the research question, "Is the job performance of nurses affected by salary or perceived job autonomy?" is (are):
   *a. Job performance
   b. Salary
   c. Perceived job autonomy
   d. Both salary and perceived job autonomy

8. The independent variable in the research question, "What is the effect of noise levels on postoperative pain or blood pressure fluctuations in ICU patients?" is:
   a. Blood pressure
   b. ICU patients
   *c. Noise levels
   d. Postoperative pain

9. The independent variable in the hypothesis, "Baccalaureate degree–prepared nurses will practice more rehabilitative nursing measures on a client in an ICU than will associate degree–prepared nurses" is:
   a. Associate degree–prepared nurses
   b. Baccalaureate degree–prepared nurses
   c. Rehabilitative nursing measures
   *d. Type of educational background of nurse

10. The purpose of an operational definition in a quantitative study is to:
    a. Assign numeric values to variables
    *b. Specify how a variable will be defined and measured
    c. State the expected relationship between the variables under investigation
    d. Designate the overall plan by which the data will be collected

11. Which of the following is a datum from a quantitative study of the labor and delivery experiences of women over age 40?
    a. Length of time in labor
    *b. 107 oz
    c. Infant's Apgar score
    d. Vaginal versus cesarean delivery

12. Which of the following is a datum from a qualitative research study on the labor and delivery experiences of women over age 40?
    a. 14.6 hours in labor
    b. 60-minute interviews one day after delivery
    *c. "It was a lot more painful than I ever imagined."
    d. 15 primiparous women with vaginal deliveries

13. For which of the following pairs of variables is there most likely to be a relationship that could be described as causal?
    *a. degree of physical activity–heart rate
    b. stress–coping style
    c. age–health beliefs
    d. parity–postpartum depression

14. A researcher's expectations about the outcomes of a quantitative study are generally expressed in the form of a:
    *a. Hypothesis
    b. Theory
    c. Dependent variable
    d. Research problem

15. The overall plan developed by the researcher to obtain answers to the questions being studied is called the:
    a. Coding plan
    b. Proposal
    c. Problem statement
    *d. Research design

16. The individuals who provide data in a research investigation are collectively referred to as the:
    a. Research producers
    b. Population
    *c. Sample
    d. Assistants

17. The following are all examples of data collection sources *except*:
    a. Self-reports
    *b. Literature reviews
    c. Observations
    d. Physiologic measures

18. Control techniques are introduced in a quantitative study as part of the:
    a. Sample selection
    b. Data Collection
    c. Data analysis
    *d. Research design

19. At what point does a qualitative researcher typically make a lot of decisions about data collection and the research sample?

a. While reviewing the literature

*c. While the study is in progress in the field

b. During the development of a research proposal

d. After a pilot study has been conducted

20. Nurses disseminate research results in:

a. Research designs

c. Literature reviews

*b. Research reports

d. Research proposals

TRUE/FALSE

(T)   1. The term *subject* is used primarily in quantitative research.

(F)   2. Quantitative researchers focus on concrete concepts, while qualitative researchers study abstract constructs.

(F)   3. Body temperature is an example of a constant.

(T)   4. Body weight is more heterogeneous among all adults living in Boston than it is among Bostonians who belong to a weight-loss program.

(F)   5. Body temperature could be a dependent variable, but not an independent variable.

(T)   6. Blood pressure is an example of a continuous variable.

(F)   7. The independent variable is the one that the researcher is interested in explaining.

(F)   8. Variables are inherently either dependent or independent.

(F)   9. In a study of the health care needs of African Americans in urban versus rural areas, race would be the independent variable.

(T)   10. An operational definition specifies the procedures and tools required for measurement of a concept.

(F)   11. In a study of the effectiveness of massage in reducing the pain of oncology patients, the researcher is investigating a functional relationship.

(T)   12. The relationship between infants' length and weight at birth is an example of a functional relationship.

(T)   13. Quantitative research typically involves a fairly linear progression of tasks.

(F)   14. The plan for converting verbal information into numeric form is known as the research design.

(T)   15. The population refers to the group to whom a quantitative researcher wants to generalize the findings.

(T)   16. In studies in which the data are collected by self-report, the people from whom the data are collected are often called the respondents.

(T)   17. If the population of interest were all RNs in the United States, a sample of nurses consisting entirely of women would not be representative.

(F)   18. The final phase in a research project is the analytic phase.

(T)   19. The progression of tasks is more linear in a quantitative study than in a qualitative study.

(F)   20. Raw data are rarely presented in qualitative research reports.

(F)   21. Qualitative and quantitative researchers always perform a literature review before collecting their data to learn what the state of the art is.

(F)   22. In a qualitative study, sample size decisions are usually determined on the basis of the number of informants available in the setting.

Reading Research Reports

■ Statement of Intent

Chapter 3 is new to this edition. It is designed to provide students early on with an understanding of the nature of research reports. It offers some practical assistance in reading research reports, with an emphasis on journal articles.

Research literature is sometimes anxiety-provoking to students because of its jargon, its dense and impersonal language, and its presentation of statistical information. Therefore, students usually need assistance in learning to read research reports—and in being persistent in their reading, even in the face of a daunting amount of new types of information. It may be helpful initially to encourage students to read research reports simply to get the gist of the report (i.e., to understand what the basic story is) without worrying about technical details. A class "translation" of a research report might be a useful exercise.

■ Selected Comments on the Research Examples in the Textbook

RESEARCH EXAMPLE FROM A QUANTITATIVE RESEARCH REPORT

White-Traut et al. (1999) prepared an abstract of their report that was included in the textbook. Here are a few comments about the abstract:

- The abstract was fairly dense and contained a considerable amount of research jargon. This is an example of an abstract that benefits from a translation (such as the one provided) to make it more accessible to an audience without extensive research skills. The translation loosens up the construction of the paragraph, replaces some technical terms with more lay terms, and uses an active voice to enliven the presentation.

- The abstract did a good job of addressing key questions. First, the researchers explained early on what the purpose of the study was: "to determine whether multisensory stimulation is safe" and leads to "improved neurobehavior and neurodevelopment."

- The abstract also clearly conveys information about the nature of the intervention: Infants in the experimental group "received 15 minutes of auditory, tactile, visual, and vestibular intervention twice a day, five days a week, for four weeks during hospitalization."

- Key aspects of the research methods are pointed out: The researchers tell readers about the population under study (preterm infants with PVL at 33 weeks post-conceptual age), the research design (a true experimental design), and the sample size (2 groups of 15 infants). Information about the dependent variables was communicated as part of the discussion of the findings.

- The abstract also succinctly summarizes a considerable amount of information about the findings. The infants in the experimental group had better outcomes than control group infants in terms of such outcomes as heart and respiratory rate and period of alertness. The absence of differences suggested that the experimental group had not suffered any injury (although with a small sample size, this would definitely require further confirmation). The intervention also resulted in cost savings.

- The researchers conclude with an overall statement about the intervention, but do not discuss the clinical implications or the study limitations.

RESEARCH EXAMPLE FROM A QUALITATIVE RESEARCH REPORT

The abstract for Kahn's qualitative study was also included in the textbook. Here are a few comments about Kahn's abstract:

- Kahn's abstract is less dense than the abstract by White-Traut and colleagues, which is commonly the case for qualitative reports. Nevertheless, the abstract does use some jargon that could be puzzling to novice readers. The translated version converts the ethnographic terminology to everyday terms.

- The abstract indicates that the purpose of the study is to examine the process that nursing home residents went through in adapting to the dual nature of the nursing home as both a home and an institution. (This purpose could, perhaps, have been articulated a bit more straighforwardly.)

- The research methods are not as fully described as might have been the case. The researcher provides information about the fact that the study was an ethnography, and for those savvy about an ethnography, this would convey a lot of information about methods. For those less savvy, a sentence or two about data collection would perhaps have been helpful. Kahn does indicate the period of data collection (9 months) and the nature of the sample (21 informants from a nursing home for older Jewish people).

- Kahn clearly described the results as revealing the residents' adaptation process, and provides information about the key dimensions of the process.

- The abstract does not conclude with suggestions about clinical implications.

■ Answers to Selected Study Guide Exercises

A.1. c 2. d 3. b 4. a 5. c 6. e

7. d 8. b 9. c 10. e 11. b 12. d

B.1. Oral report, poster session 2. Journal articles 3. Abstract

4. Headings 5. Introduction 6. Method
7. Statistical test 8. Level of significance
9. Themes 10. Results

D.2. Kachidurian's abstract was very readable and accessible to those without training in research methods. There were very few words or concepts that could not be understood by an intelligent lay person. For example, although the research design was experimental, the words "experimental group" and "control group" were avoided without any loss of information. Kachidurian simply indicated that half the infants, at random, received the special intervention while the other infants received usual care.

Although the abstract is quite brief (only 141 words), it adequately summarized most of the main features of the study. It explained the study purpose in the very first sentence. It presented information about the research methods—for example, the study population, the sample, and the research design. Information about how the dependent variable was measured was perhaps less complete than might be desired (e.g., what type of measurements yield data on the infants' head shape). The results of the study were summarized in a single sentence that corresponded to the stated intent of the study. Finally, the abstract concluded with statement about the potential implications of the findings, warning, however, that the study should be replicated for further corroboration.

■ Test Questions and Answers

MULTIPLE CHOICE

1. Nurses are most likely to find research results in:
   a. Poster sessions
   *b. Journal articles
   c. Textbooks
   d. Dissertations

2. When a research report undergoes a "blind" review, it means that:
   a. The journal editors do not know who submitted the report.
   b. The authors of the report do not know who the editor of the journal is.
   c. The report is published without indicating the authors' names.
   *d. The reviewers making recommendations about publication do not know who the authors are.

3. "New style" abstracts in research reports:
   a. Are usually no longer than 200 words
   b. Are written in paragraph style without subheadings
   *c. Appear in the journal *Nursing Research*
   d. All of the above

4. In a quantitative research report, a review of prior research on the problem under study is most likely to be found in the
   *a. Introduction
   b. Method section
   c. Results section
   d. Discussion section

5. In which section would the following sentence most likely appear: "The study sample consisted of 35 mother-infant pairs from an inner-city neighborhood."
   a. Introduction
   *b. Method section
   c. Results section
   d. Discussion section

6. In which section would the following sentence most likely appear: "The results may have been influenced by the patients' realization that they were participating in a scientific study."
   a. Introduction
   b. Method section
   c. Results section
   *d. Discussion section

7. When a finding is statistically significant, it:
   a. Suggests that the finding is very important
   *b. Has a high likelihood of being valid and replicable
   c. Proves that the researcher's hypothesis is correct
   d. Indicates the need for changes in nursing procedures

8. In which section of a research report would the following sentence most likely appear: "Patients who coughed were significantly more likely to have spontaneous dislodgement of small-bore nasogastric tubes than patients who did not."
   a. Introduction
   b. Method section
   *c. Results section
   d. Discussion section

9. In a qualitative research report, the thematic analysis of the data would be presented in the:
   a. Introduction
   b. Method section
   *c. Results section
   d. Discussion section

10. In a research report, limitations of the study are normally discussed in the:
    a. Introduction
    b. Method section
    c. Results section
    *d. Discussion section

TRUE/FALSE

(T)   1. Peer reviewers of a nursing research report are usually nurse researchers.

(F)   2. In a poster session, the researcher makes an oral report to a group of conference attendees, using the poster to illustrate key findings.

(F)   3. An abstract of a research study is generally the last section of a research report.

(T)   4. Traditional abstracts are single-paragraph summaries of the key features of a study.

(T)   5. In a quantitative study, the theoretical framework is usually described in the Introduction.

(F)   6. The research hypotheses to be tested generally are presented in the Results section, together with the statistical tests of those hypotheses.

(T)   7. The method section of a research report generally includes information about the research sample and the data collection procedures.

(F)   8. If results are statistically significant, it means that the findings are clinically important.

(F)   9. Beginning research consumers often have difficulty in reading research reports primarily because they have an insufficient knowledge base on the topic under investigation.

(F)   10. A research synopsis is another term for a research critique.

Understanding the Ethics of Nursing Research

■ Statement of Intent

The purpose of Chapter 4 is to familiarize students with the basic principles involved in the protection of the rights of humans in research. Humans are the study participants in most nursing studies, and it is important for students to understand the need to conduct such research ethically. It is also important to understand, however, that the need to adhere to ethical guidelines sometimes conflicts with the basic aim of conducting rigorous research. Therefore, instructors need to devote attention to various ethical dilemmas in which competing demands on the researcher (and on the nurse) must be balanced. An important concept in this regard is the risk/benefit ratio. Because many nurse researchers study vulnerable groups, students need to develop special sensitivity in evaluating the ethical aspects of studies involving vulnerable subjects.

■ Selected Comments on the Research Examples in the Textbook

RESEARCH EXAMPLE FROM A QUANTITATIVE STUDY

Some comments regarding the ethical aspects of Mikhail's (1999) study are as follows:

- The risks in this study could be described as minimal; although the interview might have reminded some of the respondents about stressful experiences they had had during their pregnancies, it was unlikely to be unduly stressful and might even have been therapeutic for some women because the interview provided opportunities for discussing concerns. Thus, the risk/benefit ratio seems acceptable.
- The researcher sought to reduce stress by having an African American woman conduct the interviews and recruit the sample.
- The article does not indicate whether a stipend was paid to the research subjects. If a large stipend was paid to these low-income women (which is not likely), it could be argued that the researchers used financial "pressure" to secure cooperation.

- Informed consent appears to have been properly obtained from participants.
- The researcher sought and obtained approval from an Institutional Review Board. The IRB would undoubtedly have been provided with more detail about the ethical aspects of the study than could have been included in the journal article.

RESEARCH EXAMPLE FROM A QUALITATIVE STUDY

Some comments regarding the ethical aspects of the qualitative study by Wackerbarth (1999) are presented here.

- This study posed a number of ethical challenges because of the content of the interviews. The researcher appears to have dealt with ethical issues in a thoughtful manner. Moreover, the researcher did an excellent job of communicating procedures used with human subjects to readers of the report.
- By receiving the preinterview questionnaire through the local Alzheimer's Association (with a cover letter from the director), prospective respondents were given some measure of assurance that the study was considered worthwhile.
- The researchers undertook proper steps to ensure that respondents were aware of what the study entailed. The study goals and methods were explained both in writing and orally.
- Participation in the study was voluntary: Only those who returned their preinterview questionnaire and consent form were included in the study. Informed consent appears to have been appropriately obtained.
- The researcher undertook many critical steps to safeguard the informants' privacy—an issue that is especially important in a qualitative study because the risk of identifying individual participants is greater than in a quantitative study.
- The researcher showed respect for the participants by allowing them to review, comment on, and approve written materials (including excerpts from the interview) prior to publication.
- The report did not indicate what steps were taken with the 52 people who agreed to participate in the study by completing a preinterview questionnaire, but who were not selected to be interviewed. Presumably, these individuals were appropriately informed about why they were not selected.
- The report does not indicate that the study protocols were approved by an IRB, and presumably this did *not* happen, because the report has a thorough discussion of human subjects issues. However, the protocols may have been scrutinized by the director of the Alzheimer's Association chapter, who prepared the cover letter recruiting volunteers.

▪ Answers to Selected Study Guide Exercises

A.1. d   2. b   3. c   4. b   5. a   6. d   7. b   8. a   9. c   10. a
11. b   12. d

B.1. Dilemmas   2. Nurenberg code   3. *Belmont Report*
4. Harm   5. Minimal risks   6. Self-determination
7. Full disclosure   8. Anonymity   9. Vulnerable
10. Institutional Review Boards

D.2.   Fenton and Hammond's study presents a dilemma from an ethical point of view. The most fundamental problem is that the study participants were not really given an opportunity to give their informed consent, and the intent of the researchers was not fully disclosed to people before they volunteered to participate. Indeed, the researchers deliberately deceived the participants regarding the purpose of the study. Their rationale was that deception was necessary to observe the students' natural handling of an emergency situation. If they had been told that the study concerned their reactions in a crisis, their behavior would probably not have been spontaneous, and the results would probably have been meaningless. In other words, if informed consent had been obtained, the study might not have yielded useful information.

Some people might argue that it would have been preferable simply to *observe* nursing students' reactions in a setting in which crises might occur so that deception would not be necessary. There are three difficulties with such an approach, however. First, the incidence of crises in such a setting might be relatively low, so that a great deal of time would be needed to observe 100 such situations. Second, not all crises are the same; in a natural setting, the researcher would lose control over the stimulus designed to elicit the nursing students' behaviors. Finally, in a natural setting, the behaviors of others would contaminate the participants' behaviors. Students might be relatively passive knowing that more experienced personnel were available.

In the present situation, the use of deception might, therefore, be justified. Although the students themselves probably did not derive much personal benefit from their participation (except the receipt of a $10 stipend), neither is it likely that they suffered any physical or psychological harm. It appears as though they were treated equitably, their privacy was protected, and the researcher demonstrated courtesy to them by promptly debriefing them at the end of the study. Moreover, the results of the study might be of considerable importance in curricular improvements for nursing students or in helping nurse administrators to make effective staffing decisions. On balance, the risk/benefit ratio seems acceptable.

Fenton and Hammond could be more confident that their research was ethically acceptable by conducting a small preliminary study (e.g., with 10 or so students). They could then question these students afterward and ask about their reactions to the deception and method of data collection. They could also ask them whether they would have been willing to participate even with full knowledge of what the research entailed. Fenton and Hammond should, in any event, be careful to have all aspects of the research reviewed by an appropriate human subjects committee or Institutional Review Board, or by external reviewers if such a formal committee is not available.

■ Test Questions and Answers

MULTIPLE CHOICE

1. The Tuskegee Syphilis Study violated which of the following ethical principles?
   a. Freedom from harm
   b. Right to self-determination
   c. Right to fair treatment
   *d. All of the above

2. The regulations affecting the ethical conduct of research sponsored by the federal government were incorporated into:
   a. The Nuremberg Code
   b. The Declaration of Helsinki
   *c. *The Belmont Report*
   d. The Code of Ethics of the American Nurses Association

3. Debriefing sessions are:
   a. Discussions with prospective participants before a study to obtain informed consent
   *b. Discussions with participants after a study to explain various aspects of the study and provide a forum for questioning
   c. Discussions with a human subjects committee before a study to obtain permission to proceed
   d. None of the above

4. All the following are potential benefits from participating in a study *except:*
   a. Monetary gains
   b. Access to a new and potentially beneficial treatment
   c. Opportunity to discuss personal feelings and experiences with an objective listener
   *d. Opportunity to collaborate on a study

5. The three primary ethical principles described in this chapter include all of the following *except:*
   a. Beneficence
   b. Respect for human dignity
   *c. Informed consent
   d. Justice

6. If a researcher unobtrusively studies interactions among patients in a psychiatric hospital, which ethical principle may be violated?
   - a. Confidentiality
   - b. Freedom from harm
   - *c. Right to self-determination
   - d. All of the above

7. The safeguard mechanism by which *even* the researcher cannot link the participant with the information provided is called:
   - a. Confidentiality
   - *b. Anonymity
   - c. Informed consent
   - d. Right to privacy

8. Confidentiality of study participants can be increased by:
   - *a. Avoiding the collection of any identifying information
   - b. Avoiding introducing the participants to any of the research personnel
   - c. Placing all identifying information on computer files rather than manual files
   - d. All of the above

9. Vulnerable subjects would include:
   - a. Women hospitalized for a mastectomy
   - b. Members of a senior citizens group
   - c. People who do not speak English
   - *d. Pediatric clients

10. Informed consent is not obtained when:
    - a. The researcher pays the subjects a stipend
    - *b. The researcher collects information covertly
    - c. The risk/benefit ratio is low
    - d. The researcher's study is determined to be exempt from IRB review

11. In a qualitative study that involves multiple contacts between the researcher and study participants, the researcher may negotiate a(n):
    - a. Informed consent
    - b. Stipend
    - *c. Process consent
    - d. Risk/benefit ratio

TRUE/FALSE

(F)   1. There is never any justification for violating the three primary ethical principles articulated in the Belmont Report.

(F)   2. The last major transgression of ethical principles in the conduct of research occurred in the experiments conducted by the Nazis.

(T)   3. Ethical dilemmas are inevitable in the conduct of scientific research.

(T)   4. On evaluating a study's risk/benefit ratio, consumers should weigh costs and benefits to subjects and to society.

(T)   5. The principle of self-determination concerns whether participation in a study was coerced.

(F)   6. Freedom from harm and the right to privacy are the two princi-ples on which informed consent is based.

(F)   7. Guaranteeing confidentiality to study participants means that the researcher could never link the data gathered to the person who supplied the data.

(T)   8. Observations through a one-way mirror may undermine a par-ticipant's right to full disclosure.

(T)   9. From a research standpoint, a person who does not have the competence to give his or her informed consent is considered a vulnerable subject.

(F)   10. An Institutional Review Board reviews the scientific merits of completed research.

PART II

Preliminary Steps in the Research Process

Scrutinizing Research Problems, Research Questions, and Hypotheses

■ Statement of Intent

Chapter 5 discusses methods of articulating and communicating information about the research problem via statements of purpose, research questions, and research hypotheses. There is some inconsistency in research textbooks concerning the use of such terms as aims, goals, purposes, and objectives of research, and the first section of the chapter explains how these and other related terms are used in this textbook. A specific example presented in Table 5-1 should help to clarify how the terms are defined.

The chapter then describes some of the origins of research ideas and examines the process of narrowing a specific problem from a general topic of interest. The issue of problem development within the two major paradigms is described. Alternative ways of wording the problem statement are also presented, and differences between research questions and statements of purpose are discussed.

The next part of the chapter focuses on hypotheses. The chapter explains the role that hypotheses play in giving direction to a quantitative study and in explicitly communicating that direction. It argues that quantitative studies, except for those that are purely descriptive, generally profit from the development of hypotheses before data collection. The chapter also describes the characteristics of workable hypotheses and provides guidance for a critical evaluation of hypotheses appearing in research reports. Since the wording of hypotheses is often problematic to students, considerable attention is paid to the issue of alternative wordings. The important point is that hypotheses must make predictions about the *relationship* between two (or more) variables.

■ Selected Comments on the Research Examples in the Textbook

RESEARCH EXAMPLE OF A QUANTITATIVE STUDY

Lindgren and her colleagues (1999) studied grief among the caregivers of dementia patients. Here are some comments relating the researchers' study purpose and research questions:

- The statement of purpose indicated the research variables—patterns of grief on the one hand and caregivers' experiences and losses on the other. These variables were operationally defined later in the report. The statement of purpose also specified the study population: caregivers of family members with dementia.

- The statement of purpose suggested, through the use of the verb "to determine," a focused study that would use precise, quantitative methods of data collection. This is consistent with the actual conduct of the study.

- The research problem has clearcut clinical significance. The scope of the study was manageable, and the problem was both researchable and feasible.

- The six research questions were well worded. Each one specified the variables of interest, more precisely than had been the case in the overall statement of purpose.

- The research questions flowed directly from the statement of purpose and clarified the researchers' study goals.

- The researchers did not specify explicit hypotheses. They did, however, use statistical hypothesis-testing procedures, implying that there were underlying hypotheses.

RESEARCH EXAMPLE FROM A QUALITATIVE STUDY

Sherman and Kirton (1999) conducted a study of unsafe sexual behavior among men who were HIV-positive. Here are a few comments regarding the researchers' description of their study purpose:

- Sherman and Kirton focused on a topic that is of clinical importance to nursing. The scope of the study was appropriately delimited.

- The problem was well-suited to an intensive, in-depth approach that is characteristic of qualitative studies. The approach had special potential to be productive because, as the researchers noted, there was little existing research on the phenomenon of relapsing into unsafe sexual behavior.

- The researchers communicated both an overall statement of purpose, as well as more specific research objectives. The purpose statement was rather complex and wordy, and so the five research objectives helped to better communicate what the researchers' intentions were.

- Both the statement of purpose and research objectives were communicated early in the report to assist readers in understanding immediately what the study was about.

- Consistent with the fact that this was a qualitative investigation that aimed primarily to "gain a more complete understanding of the phenomenon of sexual relapse," there were no research hypotheses being tested. However, it should be noted that other researchers might well develop hypotheses about sexual relapse based on Sherman and Kirton's findings, and test those hypotheses in a new study.

■ Answers to Selected Study Guide Exercises

A.1. 1. b   2. c   3. a   4. b   5. a   6. c   7. b   8. a

A.2. 1. a   2. c   3. d   4. a   5. b   6. d   7. a   8. c

9. b   10. d   11. b   12. c   13. b   14. a   15. c

B.1. Research problem   2. Research question   3. Research aims, objectives

4. Experience, literature, social issues, theory, external sources
5. Qualitative   6. Introduction   7. Relationship
8. Two   9. Independent, dependent   10. Multivariate, complex
11. Null (statistical)

C.6.

Independent	Dependent
4.a. Type of stimulation (tactile versus verbal)	4.a. Physiological arousal
4.b. Nurses versus patients	4.b. Perceived importance of physical versus emotional needs
4.c. Primary versus team nursing	4.c. Patient satisfaction
4.d. Frequency of turning patients	4.d. Incidence of decubitus ulcers
4.e. Patients' gender	4.e. Amount of narcotic analgesics administered
5.a. Prior blood donation versus no prior donation	5.a. Amount of stress
5.b. Frequency of initiating conversation	5.b. Patients' ratings of nursing effectiveness
5.c. Nurses' informativeness	5.c. Level of preoperative stress

Independent	*Dependent*
5.d. Draining versus no draining of peritoneum	5.d. Incidence of infection
5.e. Method of delivery	5.e. Incidence of postpartum depression

D. 2. Montanari's hypotheses are fairly clearly stated and are logically derived from her general research problem. There is, nevertheless, some room for improvement. The first hypothesis is the most problematic. As stated, it is not directly testable because there is no relationship to test. There is only one variable, the frequency of referring to nursing notes on patients' charts. What criteria will Montanari use to determine what is infrequent? It would have been more appropriate to drop the first hypothesis and to state that, in addition to testing the other hypotheses, one of the purposes of the study was to *describe* the frequency with which nursing notes are reviewed by hospital personnel. Alternatively, the first hypothesis could have been modified to make a relational prediction (e.g., nursing notes are referred to less frequently than physicians' notes).

The remaining four hypotheses are testable: All call for some comparison, which means that two variables are involved. The independent and dependent variables for these four hypotheses are as follows:

Hypothesis	Independent	Dependent
#2	Physician versus other hospital personnel	Frequency of referral to nursing notes
#3	Location of notes on chart	Frequency of physician referral to nursing notes
#4	Nurses' perception versus actual use	Frequency of referral to nursing notes
#5	Length of patient's stay in hospital	Frequency of referral to nursing notes

Given that the dependent variable is identical for hypotheses 2, 4, and 5, it would be possible to combine these three into one complex hypothesis, although it is not necessary to do so.

Three of the four testable hypotheses (2, 4, and 5) are directional. They predict some condition under which nursing notes would be more frequently reviewed. Only the third hypothesis is nondirectional—that is, the hypothesis does not predict *where* the nursing notes should be located to increase physicians' use of them. It is not really required that all the hypotheses to be the same, but unless there is some specific reason not to do so (e.g., inconsistent findings from earlier research relating to only some hypotheses), it makes more sense to state the hypotheses in a consistent format.

D. 4. Zilbermann addressed a research question that is well-suited to a qualitative approach—a question about how dyspnea is actually *experienced* by people who have a chronic pulmonary disorder. A quantitative approach could be used to study many aspects of dyspnea (e.g., frequency, intensity, etc.), but a qualitative approach is more appropriate for understanding how people *feel* and how they cope with their feelings.

The research question is one that is of relevance to the nursing profession. By understanding what patients are experiencing, nurses may be better prepared to offer assistance and support. In this instance, the research was also of *personal* interest to the researcher, who was an asthmatic. Many researchers, especially those who conduct qualitative inquiries, select topics in which they have a strong personal investment.

The research questions evolved over the course of Zilbermann's study. The general research problem was patients' reactions to dyspnea; the initial research question was rather vague—consistent with the limited information that was available on this topic. However, Zilbermann's research questions became more specific as she collected data and began to see patterns emerging. For example, she noticed that patients with different pulmonary patterns tended to react somewhat differently and so she made a decision to explore this in a systematic fashion. Overall, then, Zilbermann did a good job of selecting an important and interesting topic, addressing it within an appropriate paradigm, and then honing in on some aspects that were manageable within the context of an in-depth study.

■ Test Questions and Answers

MULTIPLE CHOICE

1. The research question, "What is the decision-making process among intensive care unit nurses who decide to assist terminally ill patients to die?" is:
   a. Most likely to be addressed using a quantitative approach
   *b. Most likely to be addressed using a qualitative approach
   c. Not researchable
   d. Not appropriately worded

2. Which of the following is *not* a major source of ideas for research problems?
   a. Theories or conceptual frameworks
   b. Personal nursing experience
   *c. Nursing code of ethics
   d. Nursing literature

3. The question, "Should voluntary tubal ligations be performed on women without children?" is:
   a. Insufficiently significant
   b. Unethical
   *c. Not researchable
   d. Acceptable as a research question

4. The research question, "Does maternal stress during the first trimester of a pregnancy affect the infant's birthweight?" is:
   * *a. Acceptable as stated
   * b. Not researchable
   * c. Not ethical for research inquiry
   * d. Not of clinical significance

5. In a research report, the statement of purpose is normally found:
   * a. In the abstract
   * b. In the first paragraph of the report
   * *c. At the end of the Introduction
   * d. At the beginning of the Method section

6. In a statement of purpose, the researcher often communicates information beyond the problem statement through:
   * a. The specification of the population to be studied
   * b. The operational definition of the research variables
   * c. The prediction of anticipated relationships among variables
   * *d. The choice of verbs that suggest the status of knowledge of the topic or the approach to be used in studying the problem

7. A research hypothesis:
   * a. Is a set of logically interrelated propositions
   * b. Is usually more general in scope than the problem statement
   * *c. Predicts the nature of the relationship between two or more variables
   * d. Predicts the absence of a relationship between two or more variables

8. The following are all purposes of the research hypothesis *except:*
   * *a. Proving the validity of a theory
   * b. Extending human knowledge
   * c. Explicating the research question
   * d. Providing direction to the research design

9. A research hypothesis indicates the expected relationship between:
   * a. The functional and causal nature of the variables
   * b. The statement of purpose and the research questions
   * *c. The independent variable and the dependent variable
   * d. Statistical testing and the null hypothesis

10. Hypotheses are:
    * a. Essential to the conduct of respectable scientific enquiry
    * b. Needed only when there is an explicit theoretical framework
    * *c. Useful in giving direction to quantitative studies
    * d. Not appropriate for most nursing research studies

11. The hypothesis, "Women who jog regularly are more likely than those who do not to have amenorrhea" is:
    - a. Null
    - b. Not correctly worded
    - *c. Directional
    - d. Nondirectional

12. A hypothesis that makes an absolute (as opposed to relative) prediction is not:
    - *a. Testable
    - b. Researchable
    - c. Justifiable
    - d. Significant

13. Hypotheses derived from a theory are almost always:
    - a. Null
    - b. Simple
    - c. Complex
    - *d. Directional

14. The hypothesis, "A person's emotional status is not affected by a relocation to a nursing home" is:
    - *a. Null
    - b. Not correctly worded
    - c. Directional
    - d. Nondirectional

15. The hypothesis, "Women who live in rural areas are unlikely to practice breast self-examination" is
    - a. Null
    - *b. Not correctly worded
    - c. Directional
    - d. Nondirectional

16. Which of the following is an example of a complex hypothesis?
    - a. Younger nurses are more likely to hold favorable attitudes toward unionization of nurses than are older nurses
    - b. The greater the amount of reinforcement a new father receives from his wife, the greater the number of functional activities he will perform for the newborn
    - c. Clinical specialist nurses perceive they have more job autonomy in the hospital than do staff nurses
    - *d. None of the above

TRUE/FALSE

(T)   1. A research problem is a situation involving an enigmatic or disturbing situation amenable to disciplined inquiry.

(F)   2. Qualitative researchers begin with a formal research question and then develop hypotheses to be tested while in the field.

(F)   3. Any question to which an answer is desired is suitable to study through systematic research methods.

(T)   4. A set of research question for a quantitative study specify the major variables in the study and the population being studied.

(F)   5. All research reports provide a clear purpose statement to guide the reader's understanding of what was studied.

(T)   6. Hypotheses in research reports are typically presented as research hypotheses rather than as null hypotheses.

(F)   7. Hypotheses derived from theory are generally nondirectional in wording.

(F)   8. Hypotheses are more abstract than purpose statements.

(T)   9. Qualitative research almost always proceeds without hypotheses.

(F)   10. Support for a researcher's hypothesis provides proof of the worthiness of the theory from which the hypothesis has been deduced.

(T)   11. A simple hypothesis states the expected relationship between one independent variable and one dependent variable.

(F)   12. Hypotheses must express the expected relationship among at least three variables.

(T)   13. The following is a null hypothesis: "Women who smoke are as likely to have low birthweight babies as women who do not."

(T)   14. The following is a directional hypothesis: "The fewer social supports an elderly person has the more likely he or she is to be institutionalized."

Reviewing the Research Literature

■ Statement of Intent

Chapter 6 describes literature reviews that are conducted within a research context. A particularly important point in this chapter is the distinction between the kind of library work that is characteristic of many nursing courses and the critical and objective appraisal of relevant research that is characteristic of a research review. Many students find this distinction difficult to grasp.

An early section of this chapter provides assistance to students in locating research reports on a specific topic. The focus is on acquainting students with available bibliographic resources, with an emphasis on electronic database searches. Hands-on exercises in the library are likely to prove helpful here.

Chapter 6 also discusses the preparation of written literature reviews. Note, however, that we do *not* include the preparation of a written review that critically evaluates the research literature as an explicit student objective for this chapter. This is because the chapter teaches some of the mechanics of doing a literature review, but it is premature at this point to expect students to critically evaluate the research literature. This skill should improve as students progress through the remainder of the textbook. We believe, however, that an understanding of what it takes to write a good research review will enhance the students' ability to appraise the literature review sections of research reports.

■ Selected Comments on the Research Example in the Textbook

RESEARCH EXAMPLE FROM A QUANTITATIVE RESEARCH REPORT

Lauver, Baggot, and Kruse (1999) prepared a brief review of the literature on women's reactions to abnormal Pap results. Here are a few comments about their literature review.

- It is, of course, difficult to know if all relevant studies were cited by these authors without doing an independent literature search. The literature review included a great many citations, many of which were published in the early to mid-1990s, but with some citations from the 1980s. It seems likely that at least some relevant studies were conducted in the late 1990s, but were not included.

- The literature review was well-organized. The review begins with a summary of available information about women's reactions to abnormal Pap tests. The review goes on to describe knowledge about women's coping strategies. Although the literature review was brief, it supports the need for the study that the researchers undertook ("However, researchers have not asked women directly to identify the type of stressors they experience . . .").

- The authors adhered to an appropriate style for the literature review presentation. Their assertions are supported by research evidence, and their opinions are not interjected in the review.

- The researchers did not actually critically evaluate the research that has already been done. Rather, the review presents brief statement statements about the type of research that had been done, noting the dearth of information on the specific research question in which they were interested.

- This literature review was briefer than is typical in a quantitative research report. It is possible that this brevity merely reflects the state of the art of knowledge on their research topic.

EXAMPLE OF A LITERATURE REVIEW FROM A QUALITATIVE STUDY

Boydell, Goering, and Morrell-Bellai (2000) drew on the literature to frame their research on the experiences of homeless people. Here are a few comments about their literature review.

- The excerpt in the text is only a portion of these researcher's literature review. In fact, the review was rather extensive for a qualitative study. The review served to document the knowledge base about the experience of homelessness and also to develop a theoretical framework for the new study that was designed to shed new light on the homeless experience.

- The majority of references for the literature review were reasonably current—almost all from the 1990s.

- The literature review was well-written and well-organized. The researchers paraphrased findings from other studies and did not rely on quotes. However, it might have been useful for the researchers to provide some documentation early in the review regarding the homeless population, such as its size and demographic composition, as a way of bolstering their argument that "the problem of homelessness is a pressing social and health concern. . . ." It would also have been useful if the researchers had developed a clearer statement about what is already known about the homeless experience and what gaps in the literature their study hoped to fill.

- The literature is judiciously referred to in the discussion section of the report, as well as being used to set the stage in the introduction.

■ Answers to Selected Study-Guide Questions

A.1. d   2. a, b   3. a, b, c   4. a   5. b
6. d   7. a   8. a   9. b, c   10. b, c

B.1. CINAHL   2. Subject   3. Textword
4. Indexes, abstract   5. Primary   6. Research
journals   findings
7. Relevance   8. Quotes   9. Gaps
10. Critical summary   11. Tentativeness

D.1. Bokan's literature review has both strengths and weaknesses. It is fairly intelligible, reasonably well organized, and concise. It makes use primarily of research findings (rather than anecdotes or opinion articles), although it seems that more recent research (post-1995) should also have been included. Most of the author's assertions are documented with citations, although there are several statements, particularly in the first two paragraphs, for which there are no references. Also, Bokan used primary sources predominantly, although there is one instance (in the last paragraph) of a secondary reference that was probably avoidable.

For the most part, Bokan used her own words to summarize what is known about PID. Her use of Eschenbach's quote in the first paragraph is not really justified. Eschenbach's words are not so dramatic, profound, or creative that they cannot be paraphrased. Using quotes in such a situation is only a crutch to avoid abstracting, summarizing, and presenting information in one's own words.

Bokan seems relatively unsophisticated with regard to research methods. Her statement in the third paragraph regarding Westrom's "proof" that PID affects fertility suggests that she does not appreciate the limitations of the scientific method. Nowhere in her review does she criticize existing research, describe its limitations, or indicate gaps in what is known.

Bokan's summary of existing studies also fails to provide pertinent information in some instances. For example, in the first paragraph, she mentions a study by Eschenbach on the incidence of gonococcal infection. The reader would form a different impression of existing knowledge if Eschenbach's study had been based on 50 cases or 5000, yet sample size and sample characteristics are not specified. As another example, Bokan describes Westrom's study in detail, yet does not indicate whether the differences between groups were statistically significant.

In summary, Bokan's literature review may be considered a good "first draft": It is flawed, but improvable. The most serious potential problem is that the review could be inaccurate if more recent research has led to different conclusions about PID. Rewriting this draft would never solve that problem.

■ Test Questions and Answers

MULTIPLE CHOICE

1. Which of the following is *not* a purpose of a research literature review for a consumer?
    a. To identify nursing interventions that have potential for use in evidence-based practice
    *b. To identify a suitable research design
    c. To acquire knowledge about a specific topic
    d. To facilitate the development of research-based protocols

2. In an online search, a person retrieves references that are:
    a. Stored on CD-ROMs in his or her own library
    b. Stored on his or her own personal computer
    *c. Directly accessed through communication with a host computer
    d. None of the above

3. The electronic database most likely to be useful to nurse researchers is
    *a. CINAHL
    b. CancerLit
    c. Health
    d. MEDLINE

4. In conducting a subject search in an electronic database, you would most likely initiate the search by typing in:
    a. An author's name
    b. Restrictions to the search
    *c. A topic or keyword
    d. A mapping procedure

5. In an electronic literature search, the searcher does not necessarily have to know precise key words for retrieving information on a topic because of the capability known as:
    *a. Mapping
    b. Searching
    c. Restricting focus
    d. Copying

6. In using print indexes, the researcher should ordinarily:
    a. Work forward from the oldest issue to the most recent one
    *b. Work backward from the most recent issue to older ones
    c. Search for articles that summarize prior research
    d. Read the accompanying abstract to determine whether the article is pertinent to the topic

7. The type of information in which the researcher is *least* interested when doing a literature review is:
    a. How the variables of interest have been operationally defined in prior studies
    *b. Narrations of a particular author's impression of a given situation
    c. Research results
    d. What research approaches have been used to study similar problems

8. A primary source for a literature review may be defined as:
   *a. A description of an investigation written by the researcher who conducted the study
   b. A summarization of relevant research that has been conducted on the topic of interest
   c. A thesaurus that directs the reader to subject headings germane to the topic
   d. Any retrieval mechanism that helps to locate articles on the area of interest

9. Which of the following sentences *best* conforms to the generally acceptable style of a research literature review?
   a. It is known that students experience anxiety in taking a test.
   *b. Several studies have found that the Lamaze method of childbirth reduces the amount of pain medication required by mothers after delivery.
   c. It is clear that motivations can not be changed overnight.
   d. Reinforcement is necessary to maintain positive behaviors.

10. Studies that integrate results of earlier research through statistical methods are known as:
    a. Meta-synthesis
    b. Mapping study
    c. Primary study
    *d. Meta-analysis

TRUE/FALSE

(T) 1. One of the major purposes of a literature review is to ascertain what research has already been done in the area.

(T) 2. A textword search allows searchers to look for topics in text fields of records in the electronic database.

(F) 3. The CINAHL electronic database covers all published nursing studies back to the early 1900s.

(T) 4. Abstract journals summarize articles that have appeared in other journals.

(F) 5. A published literature review article would be considered a primary source for a person doing a literature review on the same topic.

(F) 6. Information from anecdotal and opinion articles is usually included in a research literature review.

(F) 7. A well-written literature review is characterized by numerous quotations from research studies.

(F) 8. Paraphrasing, rather than directly quoting from an article, is a common flaw in literature reviews.

(F) 9. A good literature review includes the researcher's opinions on the issues being investigated.

(T)   10. The literature review section should conclude with a critical evaluation of knowledge on the problem of interest.

(T)   11. "Research has suggested that cigarette smoking causes lung cancer" is an appropriately worded statement for a literature review.

(F)   12. "The HIV-epidemic has been the cause of considerable anxiety in the gay community" is an appropriately worded statement for a literature review.

Examining Theoretical Frameworks

■ Statement of Intent

Chapter 7 provides some basic information about linkages between theory and research in nursing. The chapter is designed to sensitize students to the desirability of having a research problem placed in a broad conceptual context because of its potential to enhance the meaningfulness and interpretability of the findings. However, the chapter also makes it clear that most nursing research is not conducted within the context of a theoretical framework and that the absence of a formal linkage may be appropriate.

The distinction between theories, conceptual models, and frameworks is briefly discussed, as is the distinction between classic theory and descriptive theory, and the distinction between the use of theories in qualitative and quantitative research. An overview of several specific models of nursing, as well as some nonnursing models frequently used by nurse researchers, is provided. Students are not expected to become familiar with the features of these various models (indeed, insufficient information is provided in the textbook to explicate these models adequately). Rather, a major point to emphasize is that there are alternative ways of explaining and understanding phenomena of interest to nurses, and alternative explanations can be tested in the real world through empirical inquiry.

■ Selected Comments on the Research Examples in the Textbook

RESEARCH EXAMPLE FROM A QUANTITATIVE STUDY

Renker (1999) used Orem's Model of Self-Care as the conceptual framework for her study of physical abuse and pregnancy outcomes in adolescent mothers. Several comments on this study follow.

- This is a good example of a study in which the research design and interpretation of the results flowed naturally from the conceptual framework. There is nothing contrived about the linkage between the theory and the research in this example.
- Renker explicated her hypotheses, based on Orem's model, in a useful figure (Figure 1, page 380 of the full report). According to the model, physi-

cal abuse was hypothesized to have negative effects on self-care agency, which in turn (together with social support) was hypothesized to influence the young mothers' self-care practices. The final path in the model was the hypothesized effect of self-care practices on pregnancy outcomes.

• Each of the constructs in the conceptual model (also shown in the schematic model) was fully and carefully operationalized and was consistent with the underlying model. Indeed, the instruments Renker used had been previously developed specifically to assess components of Orem's theory. This illustrates the importance of having the theory-research problem linkage in place *before* undertaking the study. With an after-the-fact linkage, key constructs are rarely operationalized in an optimal way in relationship to the theory.

• The findings from the study provided support for Orem's model as a useful framework for investigating nursing problems. Consistent with Renker's hypotheses, abuse was related to self-care agency. Both self-care agency and self-care practice were significant predictors of a key pregnancy outcome, infant birthweight.

• Laudably, Renker explicitly discussed the congruence of the findings with Orem's self-care model in the discussion section.

RESEARCH EXAMPLE FROM A QUALITATIVE STUDY

Swanson (1991) developed a descriptive theory of caring based on data from three in-depth qualitative studies. Here are a few comments about Swanson's linkages between theory and research.

• This is a good example of a descriptive theory, rather than a classic theory. Swanson's goal was to thoroughly describe the caring process, not to propose relationships between caring and other phenomena.

• Swanson's theory development is greatly enhanced by the fact that she studied caring in three distinct perinatal contexts. As a result, her theory is not restricted to a single situational context. On the other hand, she might have further strengthened her position by including contexts other than perinatal ones. Fortunately, her theory is being used as a framework by researchers working with other populations.

• This example shows how theory development progresses. Swanson first identified caring processes in the first study, confirmed and refined them in the second, and added further refinements and elaborations in the third study. By the end of the third study, Swanson was able to provide a conceptual definition of caring that could serve as a foundation for other research (as well as for other applications, such as interventions and curricular developments).

• Consistent with the approach used by qualitative researchers, Swanson offered as evidence for her descriptive theory verbatim excerpts from her study participants. These excerpts greatly enhance the reader's ability to understand the descriptive theory.

- Like all theory, Swanson's theory of caring needs to be corroborated. Swanson's presentation in and of itself offers no way to evaluate the validity of the five-step process.

■ Answers to Selected Study-Guide Questions

A.1.   1. c   2. e   3. d   4. e   5. d   6. a   7. b   8. d
A.2.   1. c   2. d   3. f   4. a   5. e   6. b

B.1. Invented (created, constructed)   2. Hypotheses   3. Framework
4. Conceptual models   5. Words   6. Person, environment, health, nursing
7. Induction
8. Health Promotion Model   9. Borrowed theories   10. Grounded

D.2.   Unlike many researchers whose research reports appear in the literature, Joyce appears to have started with a theory rather than with a research problem. That is, the research hypothesis appears to flow directly from the theory. Joyce's process in deriving the research hypothesis might have approximated the following:

- Collect readings in the general area of social learning theory.

- Collect readings of studies of health-related behaviors as they relate to social learning theory.

- Based on these readings, prepare an evaluation of social learning theory as it applies to health-related behaviors.

- Present a deduction that if social learning theory were valid, then certain predictions could be made about preventive health behaviors.

- Finally, develop the specific research hypothesis.

Joyce's finding that individuals who were more internally oriented were more likely to elect membership in a Health Maintenance Organization than externally oriented people could be easily interpreted, given the fact that the hypothesis was developed on the basis of theory. It is not always so easy to interpret one's data, but having a supported hypothesis deduced from theory lends itself to fairly straightforward interpretations. The fact that the hypothesis was supported provides further support to Rotter's theoretical formulations but, of course, does not prove its validity. Similarly, if the hypothesis had not been supported, this would not constitute proof of the theory's unworthiness, but accumulated instances of research's failure to support a theory would probably seriously undermine its utility.

In the absence of a theory, this particular research problem might never have been studied; the theory indicated a construct in predicting preventive health behaviors (locus of control) that might not have been identified based on casual observations. However, it should be noted that other conceptual models and theories (e.g., the Health Belief Model, Behavioral Decision Theory) would make similar predictions but might imply a different operationalization of the key constructs.

▪ Test Questions and Answers

MULTIPLE CHOICE

1. A set of logically interrelated propositions is associated with a:
   a. Statistical model
   b. Conceptual model
   *c. Classic theory
   d. All of the above

2. The power of theories lies in their ability to:
   a. Capture the complexity of human nature by the richness of the operational definitions associated with the variables
   b. Minimize the number of words required to explain phenomena and, thereby, eliminate semantic problems
   c. Prove conclusively that relationships exist among the phenomena studied
   *d. Specify the nature of the relationships that exist among phenomena

3. The overall purpose of a theory is to:
   a. Explain relationships that exist among variables as well as the nature of those relationships
   *b. Make scientific findings meaningful and generalizable
   c. Stimulate the generation of hypotheses that can be empirically tested
   d. Summarize accumulated facts

4. The building blocks for theory are:
   a. Propositions
   b. Relationships
   c. Hypotheses
   *d. Concepts

5. The major similarity between theories and conceptual models is that both:
   *a. Use concepts as their building blocks
   b. Use the deductive reasoning process almost exclusively
   c. Contain a set of logically interrelated propositions
   d. Provide a mechanism for developing new propositions from the original propositions

6. The Health Promotion Model would best be described as a:
   a. Descriptive theory
   b. Borrowed theory
   c. Grounded theory
   *d. Middle-range theory

7. Which of the following is *not* a central concept in conceptual models of nursing?
   a. Person
   *b. Social support
   c. Health
   d. Environment

8. The nurse-theorist Orem developed the:
   a. Uncertainty in Illness Model
   b. Health Promotion Model
   c. Adaptation Model
   *d. Model of Self-Care

9. The nurse-theorist Roy developed the:
   *a. Adaptation Model
   b. Model of Man-Living-Health
   c. Science of Unitary Human Beings
   d. Health Promotion Model

10. The nurse-theorist Mishel developed the:
    *a. Uncertainty in Illness Model
    b. Health Promotion Model
    c. Adaptation Model
    d. Model of Self-Care

TRUE/FALSE

(T)   1. Classic theories offer an explanation not only of the relationship between variables but also of the nature of the relationship.

(T)   2. Descriptive theories can involve a thorough description or classification of a single phenomenon.

(F)   3. Deductive reasoning is the basic intellectual process used in *developing* a theory.

(T)   4. Theories can never be positively proved.

(T)   5. Failure of research to disconfirm a theory increases support for the theory.

(F)   6. Grounded theory is to descriptive theory as a schematic model is to a statistical model.

(F)   7. A conceptual framework may be defined as a well-formulated deductive system of abstract formal propositions.

(F)   8. Research endeavors that are not based on theory have little utility to the nursing profession.

(T)   9. Schematic models attempt to represent reality with a minimal use of words.

(T)   10. In theory-testing research, one goal of the researcher is to rule out competing explanations for the observed relationships.

(T)   11. All studies have a framework, even though not all studies are based on a theory or conceptual model.

(T)   12. Mishel's Uncertainty in Illness Theory is an example of a middle-range theory.

PART III

Designs for Nursing Research

CHAPTER 8

Understanding Quantitative Research Design

■ Statement of Intent

Chapter 8 is a very important chapter because it introduces consumers to principles that are critical to evaluating the basic architecture of a quantitative study. The chapter presents material on various dimensions of research design and techniques of research control.

The first section of the chapter provides students with an overview of some of the fundamental features of research design in quantitative studies. The major dimensions of research design (e.g., whether there is an intervention; whether the study is cross-sectional or longitudinal) are described. An important point to reinforce here is that researchers generally have considerable latitude in designing studies, but design decisions have implications for the interpretability of the study findings.

The next few sections of the chapter explain differences between research designs in which the researcher does or does not introduce an intervention of treatment—the differences between experimental, quasi-experimental, and nonexperimental designs. These sections introduce students to several important research design issues—including manipulation and randomization. The relationship between research design and causal inference is underscored. However, the text stresses the fact that although nonexperimental research limits the researcher's ability to draw causal inferences, many research problems are simply not amenable to an experimental design.

Chapter 8 also introduces some types of quantitative research that are categorized by the purposes they serve rather than by the designs that are employed. Among the types of studies discussed are the following: surveys, evaluations, and outcomes research. In all cases, the main purpose is to acquaint students with some terms used in connection with various types of research and to present an overview of the purposes and procedures of the various approaches.

Finally, Chapter 8 also describes how quantitative studies can be designed to maximize the quality and interpretability of study results through careful control over extraneous variables. Research control over external and situational factors and over intrinsic subject characteristics is discussed. This discussion is especially important because consumers must consider what design alternatives might have strengthened a study and how believable the study findings are, given the limitations of the design. Chapter 8 also introduces the concepts of internal and external validity and points out that compromise is often needed to balance design requirements for these two criteria of study worth.

■ Selected Comments on the Actual Research Examples in the Textbook

RESEARCH EXAMPLE OF AN EXPERIMENTAL EVALUATION

York et al. (1997) conducted an evaluation of an intervention for high-risk pregnant women using an experimental design. Several comments regarding this excellent evaluation are presented below:

- York and her colleagues' evaluation was multifaceted. It encompassed an impact analysis and a cost-benefit analysis. There may well have been a process analysis component to this research as well, but if there was, it was not described in the journal article. However, the article did explain in great detail what the research protocols were for the subjects in the two groups.

- York and her colleagues used a true experimental design, which offered the highest possible evidence regarding the effects of the intervention. The design was a simple after-only design—the only design possible because maternal and infant outcomes could not have been captured prior to the intervention. The design enabled the researchers to conclude with a fair degree of confidence that the observed group differences were "caused" by the intervention. (It might be noted, however, that the intervention was complex and involved several different strategies, giving rise to a classic "black box" situation—that is, it cannot be determined whether one particular aspect of the intervention was especially beneficial, or whether the entire package contributed to its success.)

- In addition to using a strong research design, the researchers offered even further evidence of the validity of their results by comparing the experimental and control group in terms of a wide array of background variables. They found, for example, that the two groups of women were comparable in terms of age, parity, education, ethnicity, income, marital status, and gestation at entry in the study.

- The value of the study was strengthened considerably by the inclusion of cost-benefit data. Administrators contemplating the implementation of a special intervention for high-risk pregnant women would naturally be interested to learn that patient outcomes were improved. But because administrators are held accountable for budgetary matters, the finding that the intervention reduced costs is likely to be particularly appealing.

- Like many evaluations, this study can also be considered outcomes research.

EXAMPLE OF A QUASI-EXPERIMENTAL DESIGN

Pickler and her colleagues (1993) used a strong quasi-experimental design to study the effect of nonnutritive sucking (the independent variable) on bottle-feeding stress (the dependent variable) in preterm infants. Here are some selected comments regarding the design of this study:

- This study is not experimental because the infants were not randomly assigned to the two groups. (Unfortunately, the authors did not indicate why an experimental design was ruled out; presumably, there were practical constraints that made randomization unfeasible).

- Although infants were not randomly assigned to the two groups, the design is nevertheless a strong one—essentially, it is a time series nonequivalent control group design. Data were collected at multiple points in time (including before and after the nonnutritive sucking) from both the experimental group and the comparison group.

- In addition to the fact that the researchers included a comparison group of infants, they took extra care to ensure the comparability of the two groups by matching the infants in terms of important characteristics: their gestational age, birthweight, gender, and race. (Unfortunately, there is no information regarding how the matching was performed—e.g., within what ranges birthweights were matched, as an indication of the precision of the matching. The absence of significant differences on these matching variables is not totally reassuring because of the small sample size).

- Despite the absence of details about the matching, the design is sufficiently strong that the results are unlikely to be biased by extraneous variables—although we cannot rule out the possibility that extraneous variables other than those used for matching purposes were differentially distributed in the two groups and influenced the observed differences in the behavioral state. Definitive conclusions are, moreover, premature due to the small sample size and the many nonsignificant results.

EXAMPLE OF A NONEXPERIMENTAL SURVEY

Heikkilä and her colleagues (1999) conducted a longitudinal survey of male and female patients undergoing coronary arteriography (CA), in an effort to understand how their fears evolved over time. Here are a few comments regarding their study design:

- This study is clearly nonexperimental and could not have been conducted as an experiment. There were, essentially, two primary independent variables: the patients' gender and the time relative to the CA procedure. Neither time nor gender could be randomly assigned.

- The researchers were interested in the evolution of patients' fears over time. They could have studied this using a cross-sectional design by studying one group of people before the CA procedure and other groups at various points after the procedure. Their decision to use a longitudinal design was, of course, far preferable.

- The researchers were attentive to issues of internal validity and sought to control an important extraneous variable, namely patients' age. They knew from the literature that age was related to patients' fears, and they also knew that there were age differences between the men and women in their sample. To better describe true gender differences, the researchers statistically controlled age in their analyses. Note that they could have used alternative control procedures. For example, they could have restricted the sample to patients within a certain age group (homogeneity). Or they could have used matching to ensure that for every woman of a certain age there was a man of comparable age. Statistical control was, however, the best approach. The researchers also included prior CA experience as a covariate.

- Given the researchers' decision to use analysis of covariance, it is somewhat curious that they did not control for background factors other than age and prior CA for which there were gender differences (e.g., marital status, number of years of cardiac problems).

■ Answers to Selected Study Guide Exercises

A.1. 1. b   2. b   3. a   4. d   5. b
      6. a   7. d   8. a   9. b   10. d

B.1. Comparison   2. Independent   3. Treatment (intervention)

4. Systematic bias   5. Random assignment   6. Pretest (baseline measure)

7. Factorial design   8. Levels   9. Double-blind

10. Repeated measure   11. Causality (causal   12. Comparison
    (Crossover)   relationships)

13. Pre-experimental   14. Time series   15. Equal (equivalent)

16. Nonexperimental   17. Correlational   18. Independent

19. Causation   20. Retrospective   21. Case-control

22. Longitudinal   23. Follow-up studies   24. Surveys

25. Evaluation   26. Constancy   27. Protocols

28. Generalizability   29. Internal   30. Selection

31. Maturation   32. History   33. External

C.3.

a. Cannot	b. Can	c. Can	d. Cannot
e. Cannot	f. Cannot	g. Can	h. Cannot
i. Can	j. Can	k. Cannot	l. Can
m. Can	n. Cannot	o. Can	

C.4.

4.a. Nonexperimental	4.b. Nonexperimental	4.c. Nonexperimental
4.d. Both	4.e. Nonexperimental	5.a. Nonexperimental
5.b. Both	5.c. Nonexperimental	5.d. Both
5.e. Nonexperimental		

D.2. Seligman and Jolly used a time series (quasi-experimental) design to test their hypothesis that the relaxation/biofeedback intervention (the independent variable) had an effect on women's menopausal symptoms (the dependent variable). Although the design has some limitations, the researchers' collection of data over an extended time period provided some measure of protection against instability or misleading findings that might arise with data collected at only two points (before and after) in time.

One of the problems with this design is that, although there are many data collection points, they are compressed in time. If this five-week period is unusual or atypical in any respect, or if something external to the study is happening concurrent with the intervention, the results could be biased or distorted.

Another difficulty with the design is that there are too many data collection points. From a practical point of view, consider the problems involved in analyzing these data. From a methodological point of view, the multiple measurements could result in inaccurate data. For example, some subjects might get bored with the task of recording their symptoms and might not pay much attention to the information they are providing. Others might be influenced in what they report on one day by what they reported on the previous day.

Because of these concerns, a more suitable design might be recommended. For example, one design would involve eight data collection points: on four consecutive weeks before the intervention and on four consecutive weeks after the intervention. The subjects might be instructed to record symptoms each Wednesday, for example, except during the three-week intervention. The elimination of data collection during the treatment period might help prevent or minimize the Hawthorne effect, that is, biases resulting from the subject's awareness of being part of a study.

The best design, of course, would be an experiment in which a randomized group of women did not get the new intervention. Random assignment might have been unfeasible for Seligman and Jolly, but they could probably have obtained a nonrandomized comparison group, that is, women not receiving the treatment. When nonequivalent control group and time series designs are combined, the resulting design is fairly powerful.

D.4.   Reynolds's study is inherently nonexperimental. Her independent variable, social/emotional supports, cannot as currently defined be manipulated by the investigator unless some serious ethical transgressions are committed (e.g., prevention or enforcement of interaction between subjects and their kin or friends). It may, of course, be possible to design an intervention with the aim of adding to the subjects' social support networks; the effectiveness of this intervention could then be tested with an experimental design. However, this would be a different study.

The study as described is prospective in nature. Reynolds first ascertained the subjects' degree of social supports. Then, six months later, she collected information on the subjects' mental and physical health. The use of a prospective design is commendable; such a design permits the researcher to establish the sequence of events. Reynolds, however, did not capitalize on this aspect of her prospective design. We cannot really be sure that the group with low social support did not have initial health problems that could have *led* to disengagement from or rejection by friends and kin. Reynolds would have done better to collect data on her dependent variables at both data collection points and then analyze the relationship between social supports and *changes* to the measures of health and morale. This would at least have enabled her to ascertain that the subjects' social support status preceded their health status.

Even with this modification, however, there are problems in using correlational data to test cause-and-effect relationships. Three conditions are necessary to establish causality. The first, determining the existence of an empirical association, has been accomplished in this example. The second, determining that the cause preceded the effect, could be established with the changes suggested above. The third condition, however, concerns ruling out the possibility that the underlying causal mechanism is not some third factor that is correlated with both the independent and dependent variables. In experiments, this condition is satisfied because groups are (presumably) equivalent with regard to everything except exposure to the independent variable. In *ex post facto* research, many extraneous variables can confound the results if they are not controlled. In the present example, the underlying cause of the subjects' health status could be their personalities: Outgoing and trusting people may be more motivated to maintain a strong social support system *and* obtain adequate health care. Other extraneous variables that could be responsible for the observed relationship between social supports and health are marital status, age, economic circumstances, and urban/rural residence, to name only a few.

D.6.   Butcher's study of contraceptive practices among college students is a nonexperimental study that can be described as a survey. The main hypothesis concerns the effect of the students' experiences with health care personnel (the independent variable) on their birth-control practices (the dependent variable). Technically, it would be possible to manipulate the kind of treatment that health care workers provide to students in dispensing contraceptive information. However, the degree to which that experience is perceived as pleasant is a subjective judgment; thus, strictly speaking, the research problem as stated is inherently nonexperimental.

In addition to being classified as a survey, the study can also be considered retrospective in nature. Butcher collected data on a dependent variable of interest (contraceptive behavior at last intercourse) and then sought information on a presumed antecedent (experience with health care workers) retrospectively. This independent variable was found to be correlated with contraceptive behavior, leading Butcher to conclude that favorable experiences result in improved contraceptive utilization. The conclusion, though possibly accurate, is not really justified by the data. There is no way of determining whether users and nonusers of contraception were comparable before their contact with the health care personnel. It is likely that they were not. It is possible, for example, for students who are most receptive to the idea of using birth control to see their contact with health care personnel in a favorable light. Several other interpretations are also possible. To strengthen his study, Butcher would have needed to control extraneous variables (i.e., to equate users and nonusers of birth control) through matching, statistical controls, or some other method. An even stronger approach would have involved a prospective design in which students had been questioned immediately after their contact with health care personnel; then, at some later point, the respondents would have been followed up to establish contraceptive behaviors and pregnancy histories.

Butcher used a mailed questionnaire to gather his survey data rather than interviewing respondents face to face. The questionnaires yielded information about a broad range of student behaviors and characteristics. The use of a questionnaire was undoubtedly an economical procedure, but the price was a relatively low completion rate: only 48% of the students responded. Because people who respond to mail surveys are rarely a random subset of the sample, the results may be biased. For example, the respondents may systematically overrepresent or underrepresent students with unfavorable experiences with health care personnel. The advantages and disadvantages of questionnaires are discussed at greater length in Chapter 11.

Butcher's use of a survey approach seems justified, although the study might have been strengthened if it had been combined with an in-depth qualitative study that intensively examined the behaviors and experiences of students in a campus health care facility that dispensed or prescribed contraceptives.

▪ Test Questions and Answers

MULTIPLE CHOICE

1. The research design for a quantitative study involves decisions with regard to all of the following *except*:

   *a. Whether there will be a theoretical context

   b. Whether there will be an intervention

   c. What types of comparisons will be made

   d. How many times data will be collected

2. One of the functions of a rigorous research design in a quantitative study is to have control over:
   - a. Dependent variables
   - b. Independent variables
   - c. Factorial variables
   - *d. Extraneous variables

3. A true experiment requires all the following *except:*
   - a. Control
   - b. Manipulation
   - *c. Double-blind procedures
   - d. Randomization

4. When the researcher simultaneously manipulates two independent variables, the design is a:
   - a. Pretest-posttest design
   - *b. Factorial design
   - c. Repeated measures design
   - d. None of the above

5. How many hypotheses can be tested in a 2×2 factorial design?
   - a. 2
   - *b. 3
   - c. 5
   - d. 6

6. The use of a random numbers table for assigning subjects to groups eliminates:
   - *a. Selection threat
   - b. History threat
   - c. Attrition
   - d. Unnecessary manipulation

7. Which of the following must be present in quasi-experimental research?
   - a. A comparison group
   - *b. Manipulation of a variable
   - c. Matching of subjects
   - d. Randomization

8. A one-group pretest-posttest design is an example of a:
   - a. Repeated measures design
   - b. True experimental design
   - c. Quasi-experimental design
   - *d. Pre-experimental design

9. In order for a researcher to examine interaction effects, which of the following designs must be used?
   - a. A time series design
   - b. A case-control design
   - *c. A factorial design
   - d. A clinical trial

10. What feature of a nonequivalent control group design makes it quasi-experimental rather than pre-experimental?
    - a. Manipulation of the independent variable
    - b. Lack of randomization
    - *c. The use of a pretest
    - d. The use of a posttest

11. A pretest is to a posttest as:
    - a. A main effect is to an interaction effect
    - b. The independent variable is to the dependent variable
    - c. A factor is to a level
    - *d. None of the above

12. One weakness associated with ex post facto research is the:
    - a. Artificiality of the setting in which it occurs
    - b. Difficulty in linking the research to a theoretical framework
    - *c. Problem of self-selection into groups
    - d. Inability to generalize the findings beyond the sample

13. Which of the following research designs is weakest in terms of the researcher's ability to establish causality?
    - a. Experimental
    - *b. Ex post facto
    - c. Pre-experimental
    - d. Quasi-experimental

14. In an ex post facto study, as compared with an experimental study, the researcher forfeits control of:
    - *a. The independent variable
    - b. The dependent variable
    - c. The baseline variable
    - d. The extraneous variables

15. In a study in which medical diagnosis is the independent variable, an ex post facto study is essential because the independent variable:
    - *a. Is inherently not manipulable
    - b. Is ethically not manipulable
    - c. Is practically not manipulable
    - d. All of the above

16. If a researcher wanted to describe the frequency with which nursing students performed breast self-examination, the study would be classified as:
    - a. Descriptive correlational
    - b. Ex post facto
    - c. Pre-experimental
    - *d. Univariate descriptive

17. Research projects that collect data at one point in time are referred to as:
    - a. Retrospective studies
    - *b. Cross-sectional studies
    - c. Longitudinal studies
    - d. Panel studies

18. A study that followed users and non-users of oral contraceptives over a twenty-year period to determine if there were any long-term side effects would be called a:
    - a. Time series
    - b. Retrospective study
    - *c. Prospective study
    - d. Repeated measures study

19. Which of the following designs involves the use of the same subjects at several points in time?
    - a. Trend study
    - b. Cross-sectional study
    - *c. Panel study
    - d. All of the above

20. The U.S. census is an example of:
    - *a. A survey
    - b. An evaluation
    - c. An experiment
    - d. An outcome analysis

21. If a researcher wanted to determine how well a prenatal program was meeting its objectives, the type of research would be a(n):
    - a. Case-control study
    - *b. Evaluation
    - c. Pre-experimental study
    - d. Survey

22. An experimental design is most likely to be used in:
    - *a. Impact analyses
    - b. Outcome analyses
    - c. Process evaluations
    - d. Formative evaluations

23. Constancy of conditions is often enhanced through:
    - *a. Having standard written research protocols
    - b. Using a randomized block design
    - c. Maximizing the internal validity of the study
    - d. Avoiding contamination of treatments

24. Using the principle of homogeneity to control for extraneous variables has implications for:
    a. Interaction effects
    *b. Generalizability of the findings
    c. Contamination of treatments
    d. Bias in the design

25. Ways by which a researcher can control extraneous variables in an ex post facto study include all of the following *except:*
    a. Using a homogeneous sample
    b. Analysis of covariance
    c. Matching subjects
    *d. Randomization

26. The most effective method of controlling extraneous variables is by:
    a. Analysis of covariance
    b. Matching
    *c. Randomization
    d. Homogeneity

27. The researcher must know *in advance* the extraneous variables that are to be controlled for which of the following procedures?
    *a. Matching
    b. Randomization
    c. Repeated measures design
    d. None of the above

28. The threat to internal validity that occurs when external events or conditions affect one group more than another is the threat known as:
    a. Maturation
    b. Selection
    c. Testing
    *d. History

29. In a nonequivalent control group design, the most serious threat to internal validity is:
    a. Testing
    *b. Selection
    c. Maturation
    d. History

30. A study is internally valid if:
    *a. All alternative explanations of the results can be ruled out
    b. An experimental design was used
    c. A repeated measures design was used
    d. A causal relationship is confirmed

31. The sampling plan for a research study affects the study's:
    a. Replicability
    b. Interaction effects
    c. Internal validity
    *d. External validity

32. When subjects' behaviors are affected not by the treatment per se but by their knowledge of participating in a study, the generalizability of the results are limited because of the influence of the:
    a. Treatment effect
    b. History threat
    *c. Hawthorne effect
    d. Selection threat

TRUE/FALSE

(T) 1. The researcher manipulates the independent variable in experimental research.

(F) 2. The experimental treatment is the dependent variable.

(F) 3. Quasi-experimental research requires the use of a comparison group.

(F) 4. The most effective method for equalizing groups of subjects that are being compared in a study is matching.

(T) 5. The one-group pretest-posttest design is an example of a pre-experimental design.

(F) 6. The type of research that has the least controls associated with it is called quasi-experimental.

(T) 7. The pretest-posttest design collects data from subjects twice.

(T) 8. Pre-experimental, quasi-experimental, and experimental research have one common feature: manipulation.

(F) 9. Clinical trials generally use a time series design.

(T) 10. The purpose of both experimental and ex post facto research is to determine the relationships that exist between the variables of interest.

(T) 11. A researcher would choose a nonexperimental approach when ethical constraints prevented manipulation of the independent variable.

(F) 12. A case-control design is typically used in prospective ex post facto studies.

(T) 13. Univariate descriptive studies focus on analyzing each variable separately rather than analyzing the association among variables.

(T) 14. A major weakness of ex post facto research is the risk of making faulty interpretations from the results.

(F) 15. A major potential problem in an experimental study is the risk of self-selection bias.

(T) 16. A study that focused on development among preterm infants would ideally use a longitudinal design.

(F) 17. Retrospective designs are stronger in determining causal relationships than are prospective designs.

(T) 18. A survey researcher collects information about the status quo of a situation.

(T) 19. Cost-benefit analyses are often conducted in conjunction with impact analyses.

(T) 20. More than one type of research control may be used in the same study.

(F) 21. A heterogeneous sample helps to control the influence of extraneous variables in a study.

(T) 22. If there is no constancy of conditions in a study, history becomes a potential threat to the internal validity of the study.

(T) 23. The threat of mortality stems from differential attrition from groups.

(F) 24. The threat of maturation is one that applies primarily to studies involving children.

(T) 25. The major threat to the internal validity of a nonexperimental study is typically the selection threat.

CHAPTER 9

Understanding Qualitative Research Design

■ Statement of Intent

The purpose of Chapter 9 is to acquaint students with some features of research design for qualitative and multimethod studies. Research design elements for qualitative studies often evolve in the field. Nevertheless, several aspects associated with quantitative design are also of relevance in qualitative design, such as *where* the study should take place, and *how often* data should be collected. In qualitative studies, however, descriptions of the research design are often after-the-fact characterizations of what emerged in response to ongoing data collection and analysis, rather than specifications of preplanned activities designed to control the research situation.

Chapter 9 also provides a brief summary of the research traditions that have guided qualitative inquiry—traditions that have provided a foundation for numerous nursing studies. Each research tradition focuses on certain types of research question—and each has its own approach to the collection and analysis of qualitative data. Only three research traditions—ethnography, grounded theory, and phenomenology—are elaborated upon, because these are the three traditions that have been most widely used by nurse researchers.

The search for truth and meaning is at the heart of systematic inquiry, and new approaches for discovering them are constantly evolving. An emerging trend in nursing research, as well as in other disciplines, is the use of multimethod research in which qualitative and quantitative data are integrated. This chapter alerts students to the many ways in which integration can advance nursing science. The fundamental rationale for blending different approaches is that integration improves the validity and interpretability of a study. The chapter describes several specific strategies for productively combining qualitative and quantitative analyses and also reviews some of the barriers to integration. Fortunately, some of these barriers are disappearing.

■ Comments on the Actual Research Examples in the Textbook

EXAMPLE OF A GROUNDED THEORY STUDY

Sayre (2000) used the grounded theory method to study patients' explanations of their being hospitalized for a severe mental illness. The following are some comments regarding the design and conduct of this study.

- Sayre's study focused on a problem that is well-suited to a flexible design using qualitative methods. It is difficult to imagine how Sayre productively could have used a more structured research design.

- The grounded theory method, in particular, was especially appropriate given Sayre's aims. She wanted to understand the process by which psychiatric patients made sense of their hospitalization. The questions she raised were not suitable, for example, to an ethnography, which might have focused on the culture (e.g., the norms, the language, the interactions) of a psychiatric ward. Nor do the questions lend themselves to a phenomenologic inquiry, which would have focused on the lived experience of hospitalized psychiatric patients. Grounded theory studies seek to understand social processes and how these processes evolve as a result of a social experience, and this is exactly what Sayre sought to do.

- Sayre's study was strengthened by the intensity of her engagement in field work. Sayre interviewed study participants during their first week of admission and then several more times until they were discharged from the hospital. Through this approach to her field work, she was able to gather immediate, first-hand, and in-depth information about the patients' experiences and how the patients came to terms with their hospitalization.

- Her study was also strengthened by her decision to gather many different types of data (what we will describe later in the text as data source triangulation and method triangulation). As described in the full report, Sayre gathered data by interviewing people, by making observations of interactions in the hospital, and by reviewing medical records. She interviewed patients and also had discussions with staff. Her questioning evolved over the course of data collection so that she could capitalize on what she was learning, a noteworthy strength of a flexible design.

- As dictated by the methods of grounded theory, the researcher simultaneously collected and analyzed her data. Use of this method yielded rich findings in which the basic social process emerged, namely managing self-worth to deal with the stigma of being a mental patient.

EXAMPLE OF AN ETHNOGRAPHIC STUDY

Dreher and Hayes (1993) undertook an interesting and complex field study within the ethnographic tradition. Some selected comments about the design and conduct of their study follow:

- The researchers ensured that they would thoroughly understand the context of the use of ganja among Jamaican women by spending a very long period of time in the field—six years. Through such intensive, long-term study, the researchers could be relatively sure that they had been able to gain an emic perspective on the phenomena under investigation. Furthermore, by remaining in the field for six years, they were actually in a position to observe changing trends in the use of ganja among women.

- The researchers gathered a wealth of data that likely increased the validity of their findings. For the qualitative portion of their study, they interviewed many women and actively participated in their lives. They got to know not only all of their study participants, but the whole community in which participants lived.

- A very interesting feature of this research is that it combined an ethnographic study with a clinical study. Not only did the data from the two parts of the study supplement each other nicely—the work in the ethnographic study helped to form the basis for the clinical study: Through their in-depth knowledge of the culture, the researchers were better able to adapt the child assessment instruments and administer them properly.

EXAMPLE OF AN INTEGRATED STUDY—THEORY BUILDING

Connelly and her co-researchers undertook a multimethod study with the aim of refining a model to explain nurse retention. Here are a few comments on their study.

- This study was primarily quantitative. The researcher's began with the aim of developing a statistical model to explain nurse retention. They used structured instruments designed to capture factors relating to retention that were identified in the research literature, and they implemented a structured nonexperimental research design to test their model. However, unlike many research projects, the researchers pushed beyond their original design when they realized that the predictive power of their model was modest. They decided to pursue an in-depth inquiry to better understand the limitations of their model.

- This study provides an illustration of a two-step data collection process. Had the qualitative portion of the study been undertaken at the same time as the quantitative portion, the researchers might not have been able to properly frame their in-depth questions. Moreover, the researchers were able to "hand pick" respondents for the second stage who were best able to yield information about job retention—that is, nurses who stayed in their jobs despite the fact that they initially appeared unlikely to do so. (It is possible that the researchers might have gained even further insights by conducting in-depth interviews with nurses who initially appeared committed to their jobs, but who nevertheless left.)

• As the researchers so aptly noted, a multimethod approach offered several advantages, including the validation of factors already included in the model. The most important contribution, however, was the expansion of the researchers' understanding of the factors contributing to staff retention—an understanding that should prove valuable in future quantitative studies of nurse retention and in the refinement of the model.

■ Answers to Selected Study-Guide Exercises

A.1.   1. b   2. a   3. d   4. c   5. b
       6. a   7. b   8. c   9. d   10. c
A.2.   1. c   2. a   3. b   4. d   5. a
       6. c   7. b   8. c   9. c   10. a

B.1. Emergent   2. Bricoleurs
  3. Anthropology, psy- 4. Cultures
     chology, sociology
  5. Macroethnography,   6. Researcher as instrument
     microethnography
  7. Essence
  8. Spatiality, corporeality, temporality, relationality
  9. Grounded theory   10. Constant comparison
 11. Complementary   12. Qualitative, quantitative
 13. Incremental   14. Validity
 15. Instruments   16. Interpretation

C.2.   a. Grounded theory   b. Ethnography
       c. Discourse analysis   d. Phenomenology

D.2.   Methodologically, Dake and Talman's study has both strengths and limitations. The design chosen, grounded theory, was appropriate for the purpose of the study, which was to examine the process women go through over the first twelve months after relinquishing their babies for adoption. Certain aspects of the sampling design were also commendable. The women in this sample had a range of ages, were both married and single, and had made their decisions to give their infants up for adoption at different times during their pregnancies. The diversity on these important variables likely contributed to a richer and fuller array of data on which to base an emerging conceptualization of post-adoption adaptation, and also could contribute to the transferability or generalizability of the study findings. (It is unfortunate, however, that the sample was restricted to white, economically advantaged women). Moreover, it seems likely that with a sample of twenty-eight study participants, the researchers achieved some stability in the themes that emerged (i.e., that data saturation was achieved).

However, the brief summary suggests some possible limitations. First and foremost, in grounded theory studies, data collection and data analysis should occur simultaneously. New data should be constantly compared with previously obtained data. This constant comparative method is used to determine which participant is to be interviewed next (and what type of data to obtain) to best develop the grounded theory. Dake and Talman failed to carry out this critical piece of the grounded theory method. They conducted all their interviews first, and only began their analysis when all twenty-eight interviews were completed.

Another limitation of the study has to do with what is called "method slurring." In method slurring researchers combine features from different qualitative traditions into one study. Dake and Talman appear to have mixed grounded theory methods with phenomenologic methods. As a grounded theory study, the outcome of this research should have been the description of the phases or stages women went through as they resolved or coped with the basic problem of mourning the loss of their child. Instead, the researchers identified four themes describing the women's experiences. Themes are more appropriate as the outcomes for a phenomenological study.

Based on the brief description of the methods used, it appears that Dake and Talman would have had difficulty fully describing the women's process of adaptation. The interviews were fairly brief, considering the aim of discovering underlying processes. Moreover, the researchers' understanding was likely constrained by their decision to gather data only at one point in time, relying on the women's retrospective accounts of their post-adoption experiences. A longitudinal design seems much better suited to their stated purpose.

One final note is that the four "themes" appear to overlap considerably and could perhaps be more parsimoniously presented as only one or two themes. At the same time, it is somewhat surprising that all of the themes are negative—that is, that none of the themes relate to such plausible post-adoption emotions as the relief that some women may have felt about not having the responsibility for a child who, for whatever reason, was not wanted; or gratification in the knowledge that the children might experience benefits in their adoptive homes.

D.4.   Zack's main approach was quantitative—the collection of structured data by means of a survey. However, she embedded a qualitative data collection approach (unstructured interviews) within the survey. By combining strategies that yielded both qualitative and quantitative data, Zack was able to gather a rich set of data. The structured interviews allowed her to collect specific information about breastfeeding practices and duration and about specific predictors of breastfeeding, such as demographic characteristics and personal attitudes. The structured interviews also allowed her to measure a number of psychological variables using established scales whose psychometric properties were known in advance. Using sophisticated multivariate procedures, these data would allow her to "explain" and predict variation in breastfeeding status and duration.

These analyses, however, might not really allow Zack to *understand* this variation. For example, if the prediction equation indicated that teenaged mothers who did not breastfeed their babies had lower self-esteem than those who did, what does this really *mean*? *How* does low self-esteem function to inhibit breastfeeding? It is possible that the in-depth data, collected by means of an unstructured topic guide, would shed light on the meaning of the findings. It is also possible that the qualitative analyses would confirm that, in this hypothetical example, self-esteem is an important construct in teenagers' decision making relating to breastfeeding. It therefore is likely that the collection of both qualitative and quantitative data in Zack's study enhanced the validity and interpretability of the findings.

Nevertheless, it is also possible to imagine ways in which the study design and data collection effort could be further strengthened. First, it might be pointed out that Zack's decision to conduct in-depth interviews with only those teenagers who were interviewed at home was ill-advised. It is true that such in-depth interviews are not appropriate for the telephone and should have been conducted in a face-to-face situation. However, in Zack's study, all the in-person interviews were conducted with teenagers who could not be interviewed by telephone (presumably because the teenagers did not have telephones or had such irregular hours that they could not be contacted by telephone), thereby leading to a situation in which all the in-depth interviews were conducted with a biased subset of the sample. Zack should have made arrangements to conduct some in-depth interviews with telephone respondents.

Zack's study would probably also have been strengthened if the data had been collected at multiple points in time. For instance, she might profitably have begun with some in-depth interviews to understand better the nature of the breastfeeding decision. If she had done so, she might have opted for different scales and questions to be included in the structured interview. For example, the in-depth interviews might have revealed the importance of such constructs as "body image" or "cognitive maturity"—constructs that were not measured in the structured interviews at all. As another alternative, it might have been useful to postpone the in-depth interviews until after the quantitative data had been analyzed. To pursue the example suggested previously, if the multivariate analysis of the data from the structured interview had indicated that self-esteem was important in understanding breastfeeding patterns, then perhaps a large portion of the in-depth interviews could have focused on this construct. An iterative approach to multimethod research offers many advantages.

■ Test Questions and Answers

MULTIPLE CHOICE

1. The term *emergent design* in the context of a qualitative inquiry indicates that the research design emerges:
   - a. During the conduct of a literature review
   - b. While the researcher develops a conceptual framework
   - c. During the process of doing constant comparisons
   - *d. While the researcher is in the field collecting data

2. All of the following are issues that a qualitative researcher attends to in planning a study *except*:
   - a. Selecting a site
   - b. Determining how best to gain entrée in key settings
   - *c. Selecting data collection tools
   - d. Determining the maximum amount of time available for field work

3. Which of the following design features can apply to both a qualitative and quantitative study?
   - a. Manipulation of the independent variable
   - *b. Cross-sectional or longitudinal data collection
   - c. Control over extraneous variables
   - d. Random assignment of study participants

4. The research tradition known as *ethnoscience* has its roots in the discipline of:
   - *a. Anthropology
   - b. Philosophy
   - c. Psychology
   - d. Sociology

5. The research tradition known as *ethnomethodology* has its roots in the discipline of:
   - a. Anthropology
   - b. Philosophy
   - c. Psychology
   - *d. Sociology

6. The research tradition known as *hermeneutics* is closely allied to another research tradition known as:
   - a. Ethnography
   - *b. Phenomenology
   - c. Ethology
   - d. Symbolic interaction

7. Ethnographers strive to:
   - *a. Understand human cultures
   - b. Develop an etic perspective
   - c. Link the etic and emic perspectives into a unified whole
   - d. All of the above

8. Which of the following is *not* a step in the phenomenologic approach?
   - a. Bracketing
   - *b. Inferring
   - c. Analyzing
   - d. Describing

9. A researcher gets on an elevator and, instead of facing forward, faces backward toward other elevator passengers. This would be an example of:
   a. An ethnographer's attempt to gain an emic perspective
   b. A phenomenologist's effort to appreciate the essence of what the passengers are experiencing
   *c. An ethnomethodologist's attempt to understand the social expectations regarding behavior in an elevator
   d. A discourse analyst's attempt to listen to people's conversation on an elevator

10. Which of the following approaches involves the use of a procedure known as constant comparison?
    *a. Grounded theory
    b. Ethnography
    c. Phenomenology
    d. Ethology

11. "What is the essence of men's experiences of chemotherapy treatment for prostate cancer?" is an example of a research question within which of the following traditions?
    a. Grounded theory
    b. Ethnography
    *c. Phenomenology
    d. Ethology

12. "What is the basic social process women use through their menopausal transition?" is an example of a research question within which of the following traditions?
    *a. Grounded theory
    b. Ethnography
    c. Phenomenology
    d. Ethology

13. The use of both qualitative and quantitative data in a study or cluster of studies serves the important purpose of:
    a. Providing researchers with different skills and an opportunity to collaborate
    *b. Enhancing the validity of the study
    c. Allowing research subjects to select whether they prefer an unstructured or structured method of responding
    d. Enhancing the likelihood that the study will be published

14. When the qualitative and quantitative data from a single study are inconsistent with one another, this provides:
    a. Evidence that the findings are not trustworthy
    *b. An opportunity to push the line of inquiry on a topic further
    c. A situation requiring that one type of data or the other be ignored
    d. An excellent publication opportunity

15. The black box refers to:
    a. Variation in the dependent variable that the researcher cannot explain
    b. The computer programs that analyze research data
    c. The constructs of interest to researchers that have defied measurement efforts
    *d. The underlying, unmeasured causes or mediators of the observed effects of an intervention

16. Which of the following types of studies could effectively combine qualitative and quantitative methods?
    a. An experimental evaluation of a nursing intervention
    b. A follow-up study of cancer survivors
    c. A study to develop a new clinical assessment instrument
    *d. All of the above

TRUE/FALSE

(F)   1. Design decisions evolve while the study is in progress in both qualitative and quantitative studies.

(F)   2. Unlike quantitative researchers, qualitative researchers do not use group comparisons to promote understanding of phenomena of interest.

(T)   3. Qualitative researchers eschew the concept of constancy of conditions.

(T)   4. A qualitative researcher typically enters the field not knowing what is not known.

(F)   5. Qualitative studies are never prospective studies.

(F)   6. Human ethology studies the essence of human behavior through in-depth discussions with study participants.

(T)   7. Discourse analysis focuses on human communication.

(T)   8. An ethnographic study of a nursing home is an example of a microethnography.

(F)   9. The etic perspective is the "insider's view"—the way the members of a culture see the world.

(F)   10. Phenomenologists focus on the manner by which people make sense of social interactions.

(F)   11. Bracketing refers to the process of separating qualitative data from quantitative data.

(T)   12. Interpretive phenomenology stresses the meaning of human experience.

(T)   13. Constant comparison is a technique used in grounded theory in developing theoretical categories.

(F)   14. Qualitative data are more profitably integrated into studies that are basically quantitative than vice versa.

(T)   15. The validity of a study is enhanced when a hypothesis is supported by complementary types of data.

(T) 16. The use of qualitative methods as a preliminary step in the development of structured instruments is an approach to building validity into the instruments.

(T) 17. When qualitative and quantitative approaches are combined, it is often productive to use a two-stage data collection approach.

(F) 18. Most nursing research involves a multimethod approach.

Examining Sampling Plans

■ Statement of Intent

Chapter 10 introduces students to the concept of sample selection for both quantitative and qualitative studies. As in other aspects of study design, sampling issues are handled quite differently by researchers working within different paradigms in terms of goals, approaches, and criteria for evaluating sample adequacy.

With regard to quantitative research, the chapter describes several types of nonprobability and probability samples and offers guidelines for assessing the quality of the researcher's sampling approach. Detailed procedures concerning the complex topic of sample size are not discussed, but the point is emphasized that sample sizes in quantitative studies should generally be large, especially if the population is heterogeneous with respect to the variables of interest. The principles underlying a power analysis are also described, and an example is used to show that generally fairly large samples are needed to adequately test research hypotheses. The point is made, however, that size alone cannot guarantee a good sample. A sample for a quantitative study is good if it is *representative,* and several factors—most importantly, size, method of selection, response rate, and subject attrition—determine a high-quality sample. The issues of representativeness of a sample and the adequacy of sample sizes are particularly important because many quantitative nursing research studies have weak sampling designs.

Qualitative researchers employ very different strategies and are guided by different considerations than quantitative researchers. The chapter describes several alternative approaches that are used to enhance the *information-richness* of the data obtained in a qualitative study. In a qualitative study, random selection is not only not attempted, it is eschewed. Sample size is also guided by data adequacy rather than by the need to achieve certain statistical goals.

■ Selected Comments on the Research Examples in the Textbook

RESEARCH EXAMPLE FROM A QUANTITATIVE STUDY

In her study of health care workers' use of gloves, Levin (1999) used a sampling design with numerous commendable features as well as a few limitations. Below are a few comments regarding her sampling plan:

- Levin sought a sample of registered nurses and medical laboratory workers who had exposure to human blood. The sampling frame consisted of (1) all registered nurses with active registration status in Illinois and (2) medical lab workers certified through the American Society of Clinical Pathologists' Board of Registry. By having a sampling frame of the complete universe of RNs and medical lab workers in Illinois, Levin was assured that her information would not be restricted to glove use practices within a single institution, or within certain types of institutions or locales.

- Another commendable feature of the design is that Levin randomly sampled from the sampling frame, ensuring that there would be no systematic biases (except those that might arise from nonresponse).

- Levin's response rate was, for a mailed questionnaire, very respectable (69.7%). This high response rate was achieved, in part, through Levin's exemplary follow-up efforts. She mailed a reminder postcard within one week of mailing the survey, and a second copy of the questionnaire to nonrespondents three weeks later. (Note that Levin was able to identify nonrespondents, and thus it is likely that the questionnaires were not anonymous; this might have depressed response rates—but obviously not by much.)

- Levin achieved a good sample size—higher even than she determined was necessary to adequately test her conceptual model. The final sample was 527 health care workers, and the desired sample size was 450.

- A potential concern stems from the fact that Levin did not fully describe her sampling design. The report stated that she randomly sampled "by telephone area codes for Chicago, its suburbs, and the rural area of Illinois." It is not clear if any part of Illinois was excluded, and, if so, what parts and why—since the study involved a mailed questionnaire.

- The report also did not indicate whether there were any nurses or lab workers for whom a telephone number was not listed in the directories—and, if so, how prevalent this problem was. Information could also have been provided regarding (a) how recent the directories were, relative to when the questionnaires were sent; and (b) how many questionnaires were returned because sample members had moved.

- The investigator was able to analyze two types of response bias. First, she looked at whether nurses and lab workers had different response rates (they had very similar rates). Second, she examined whether response rates varied by locale, presumably based on the area codes. She learned that nurses in Chicago were significantly less likely to return their questionnaires than others. Levin did not, however, indicate the potential effect of such bias (e.g., did nurses in Chicago have different glove-use behaviors than others?) Also, Levin did not indicate whether any other type of response bias analysis could have been conducted. Clearly, complete demographic information about nonrespondents was not available but it is possible that directories provided information that could have been used in such an analysis (e.g., type of degrees).

- Overall, however, Levin's sampling plan was very strong, and the absence of certain types of information in the report could reflect space constraints rather than true omissions or oversights.

RESEARCH EXAMPLE FROM A QUALITATIVE STUDY

Ledlie (1999) used a combination of sampling strategies in her study of family caregivers' disclosure of children's HIV status. Here are a few comments regarding her sampling plan:

- Ledlie wanted to understand how families manage diagnosis disclosure to a child with perinatally acquired HIV disease. Given the purpose of her study—which did not seek to document specific facts, such as the percentage of caregivers who make such a disclosure to children at specified times in their lives—her decision to conduct a qualitative study and to use a sampling plan that would yield information richness was appropriate.

- The researcher began by purposefully selecting families who had and had not disclosed the diagnosis. Her decision to specifically include both types of families in the research seems well-founded. In order to understand how the caregivers managed diagnosis disclosure, she had to ensure that her sample would include both families who had already made the decision to disclose, as well as others still wrestling with the issue. (Of course, Ledlie could also have conducted the study longitudinally and followed families who had not yet disclosed over time. However, this would require more resources, more time, and the risk of losing families over the study period.)

- After beginning with a purposive strategy, Ledlie then used theoretical sampling. Theoretical sampling allowed her to use early information to shape her sampling in such a way that maximum utility could be gleaned from the remaining interviews. It is possible that a more elaborate sampling design (e.g., simple random sampling) might actually have done a worse job of capturing the full range of thematic content, given how small the sample size was.

- Laudably, Ledlie also sought participants who varied demographically, ensuring that the emerging theory could be maximally developed.

- The sample size of twenty families is small, but not unusually small for a grounded theory study. Unfortunately, the research report did not indicate that sample size decisions were based on data saturation. (Of course, this does not mean that saturation was *not* the guiding principle, only that this was not made explicit.)

- Ledlie's description of the sample suggests that she was successful in recruiting a heterogeneous sample of families who varied with regard to age, race, and socioeconomic status. Caregivers varied in terms of their relationship to the child and the time they had spent as caregiver. Children varied in terms of HIV serostatus, age at diagnosis, and disease stage. These are all characteristics that could affect diagnosis disclosure.

■ Answers to Selected Study-Guide Questions

A.1. 1. c   2. a   3. d   4. b   5. c
      6. b   7. c   8. d   9. a   10. d

A.2. 1. b   2. c   3. a   4. b   5. b
      6. c   7. a   8. a   9. d   10. b

B.1. Sample   2. Representativeness   3. Biased
   4. Homogeneous   5. Accidental sample   6. Strata
   7. Judgmental; purposeful; theoretical   8. Simple random
                                                    sampling
   9. Weighting   10. Multistage   11. Sampling interval
  12. Sampling error   13. Accessible   14. Increases
  15. 30   16. Information
  17. Maximum variation 18. Typical case

C.2. a. Cluster   b. Convenience   c. Systematic
         (multistage)
      d. Quota   e. Simple random   f. Snowball (network)

D.2.   Dolan's sampling design can best be described as quota sampling. She
had the names of students from three types of nursing programs[1] and used essentially sampling by convenience to fill 100 slots for each type. Dolan's sampling design has some good features. In particular, her selection of 100
students from the three programs guaranteed that all three types would be
adequately represented in the survey. Her procedure was thus better than it
would have been had she merely obtained the lists and then surveyed the first
300 students she could locate.

Dolan's method of obtaining respondents for each of her three cells, however, exposed her to a considerable risk of bias. Given that local telephone directories were used to locate subjects, it is highly probable that certain
students were automatically excluded from the sample. Students who had
moved from the area, had unlisted phones, had changed their surnames, or
had phones listed under roommates' names had no opportunity to be included in the study. Such students probably differ systematically from students who *were* accessible through telephone directories. For example,
students who had moved from the area might consist of a disproportionately
high percentage who got good job offers, who got no job offers, or who decided to go to graduate school. There is no way of knowing the nature and
extent of the biases in Dolan's sample.

Several steps could be taken to improve Dolan's design. She would probably have had better success in locating graduates had she sought the cooperation of either the nursing schools or the state licensing agency. Another

---

[1]Schools were selected according to a quota system with two per site.

alternative would have been to contact students before graduation and obtain their address or the name and address of a person through whom they could be contacted, such as a parent or sibling. If these steps had been taken, Dolan might have been able to select a random sample of graduates.

If Dolan could not follow the above suggestions for some reason, she could still have introduced somewhat more control into her design. For example, she could have selected a random sample of 100 students from each program type and then made a more concerted effort to locate the selected graduates. She could have asked for leads or contact information from the students she *was* able to locate, or she could have inaugurated a postal search by mailing a letter to prospective participants at the school of nursing.

Even modest adjustments would have been likely to improve the representativeness of the final sample. It would probably have been relatively easy to introduce additional strata into the sampling design. Then, even with accidental sampling within strata, according to a quota system, some biases might have been eliminated or reduced. Examples of other strata about which information could have been obtained from either the nursing school or prospective respondents include gender, field of specialization, and whether the subject was an honors student.

The abstract did not specify Dolan's target and accessible populations. It is probably safe to assume that her accessible population was recent nursing graduates residing in the greater Boston area. The most conservative definition would be that the accessible population consisted of graduates of six Boston-area nursing schools residing in or near Boston with a published telephone number. It would take a giant leap of faith to assume that these 300 subjects adequately represented the target population of recent nursing graduates in the United States, as implied.

Dolan's sample size is modest for a survey of this type because one would expect considerable diversity (heterogeneity) with respect to job-seeking experiences. Still, 300 is a fairly respectable number and is probably adequate for most purposes. If Dolan had taken steps to improve the representativeness of the subjects, her sampling approach probably would have been acceptable.

One final consideration involves Dolan's stratification. Her plan involved the use of disproportionate sampling (i.e., 100 may be a 10% sample of baccalaureate students from the two schools but a 30% sample of diploma students from the two diploma schools). Given the probability that Dolan's sample is not representative of the target or accessible populations, it is somewhat irrelevant whether proportionate or disproportionate sampling was used. If she had been able to obtain a stratified random sample through a method such as that described earlier, a proportionate sampling design would probably have been the best way of obtaining accurate estimates of population values.

D.4.   Lombardo began with two purposive samples of couples who had fertility impairments—those who had and those who had not (yet) achieved a pregnancy. Within each group, Lombardo sought to maximize variation with regard to several aspects of the fertility problem and its treatment.

By using a maximum variation approach, Lombardo was able to get a handle on the breadth of issues that related to these couples' quality of life. Based upon what she learned from the initial five or six interviews, Lombardo then sought couples whose experiences had the most potential to achieve data saturation on the themes that had emerged. Had Lombardo planned her sampling strategy in advance, she might have missed some opportunities to enrich her data in theoretically important ways.

It is unclear from the brief summary whether the total sample size of twenty couples was adequate. However, since sampling decisions were guided by the desire for data saturation, one must assume that the researcher was successful in achieving it.

■ Test Questions and Answers

MULTIPLE CHOICE

1. Sampling may be defined as the:
   a. Identification of the set of elements used for selecting study participants
   *b. Process of selecting a subset of the population to represent the entire population
   c. Aggregation of study participants who meet a designated set of criteria for inclusion in the study
   d. Technique used to ensure that every element in the population has an equal chance of being included in the study

2. Bias in a sample for a quantitative study refers to:
   a. Lack of heterogeneity in the population on the attribute of interest
   b. Sample selection in nonprobability-type sampling
   c. The margin of error in the data obtained from samples
   *d. Systematic over- or underrepresentation on the attribute of interest vis-a-vis the population

3. Strata are incorporated into the design of which of the following types of samples:
   a. Systematic
   b. Purposive
   *c. Quota
   d. Simple random

4. Nonprobability sampling includes all the following *except*:
   a. Convenience sampling
   *b. Cluster sampling
   c. Purposive sampling
   d. Quota sampling

5. Of the following, the type of sampling design that would be especially likely to yield a representative sample is:
   *a. Systematic
   b. Convenience
   c. Purposive
   d. Quota

6. Of the following types of sample, which one is considered to be the weakest for quantitative studies?
   *a. Convenience   c. Purposive
   b. Quota   d. Systematic

7. The type of nonprobability design that is most likely to yield a representative sample is:
   a. Convenience sampling   *c. Quota sampling
   b. Purposive sampling   d. Network sampling

8. The procedure of weighting is associated with which type of sampling design?
   a. Proportionate sampling   c. Simple random sampling
   *b. Disproportionate sampling d. Quota sampling

9. A researcher used a probability-type systematic sampling plan. The sample size was 200. The sampling interval was 250. The first element drawn was 196. The second element would be:
   a. 396   *c. 446
   b. 450   d. 646

10. A researcher used a systematic sampling design. The known population size is 3200, and the desired sample size is 160. What is the sampling interval?
    a. 16   c. 160
    *b. 20   d. 320

11. Which of the following terms does not belong with the others?
    a. Purposeful sample   c. Theoretical sample
    b. Purposive sample   *d. Volunteer sample

12. Theoretical sampling is primarily concerned with adequate representation of:
    a. Sampling units   c. The target population
    *b. Themes   d. The accessible population

13. In a qualitative study, sample size decisions are often guided by the principle of:
    a. Emergent theory   c. Representativeness of informa-
    *b. Data saturation   tion
                             d. Sample diversity

14. As a qualitative researcher nears the end of data collection, he or she may employ the technique of sampling:
    a. Critical cases   c. Typical cases
    b. Deviant cases   *d. Disconfirming cases

TRUE/FALSE

(F)   1. Sampling bias would be of greater concern in studying body temperatures in healthy adults than in studying their attitudes toward abortion.

(T)   2. The major criterion in assessing the adequacy of a sample in a quantitative study is the degree to which it represents the characteristics of interest in the population.

(T)   3. Random selection is used in all types of probability sampling designs.

(F)   4. If a probability sampling design has been used, the researcher can safely generalize to the target population.

(F)   5. Systematic sampling involves the successive random sampling of units from largest to smallest.

(T)   6. In a quantitative study, larger samples are more likely to represent the population on the attribute of interest than smaller samples.

(F)   7. Snowball sampling is to convenience sampling what cluster sampling is to simple random sampling.

(F)   8. Each element in the population has an equal chance of being selected in a quota sampling plan.

(T)   9. Systematic sampling may be of a probability or nonprobability nature.

(F)   10. The researcher hand-picks people to be included in a study in cluster sampling.

(F)   11. Differences between population values and sample values are referred to as weighting errors.

(T)   12. Power analysis is used to estimate the sample size needed to adequately test research hypotheses.

(T)   13. In a quantitative inquiry, populations that are homogeneous with respect to the dependent variable require a smaller sample size.

(F)   14. A major criterion for assessing the adequacy of a sample in a qualitative study is the degree to which a theory has been developed to adequately describe the population.

(T)   15. Qualitative researchers often strive to purposefully select sample members based on emerging information needs.

PART IV

Collection of Research Data

Scrutinizing Data Collection Methods

■ Statement of Intent

Chapter 11 describes the major methods of obtaining research data. After an introductory section that discusses the use of existing data versus the gathering of new data, the text goes on to explain that methods of gathering data differ on four critical dimensions (structure, quantifiability, researcher obtrusiveness, and objectivity) and in basic approaches (self-report, observation, biophysiologic measure). It is important for consumers to understand how much flexibility a researcher has in operationalizing variables and to realize that the decisions that the researcher makes should be subjected to critical scrutiny.

The chapter then describes the major features of the primary forms of data collection used by nurse researchers, namely self-reports, observational techniques, and biophysiologic measures. Structured forms of data collection amenable to quantitative analysis as well as unstructured forms of data collection amenable to qualitative analysis are described.

The section on self-reports discusses various forms of unstructured self-report techniques, such as focused interviews, life histories, and focus group interviews. With respect to more structured self-report techniques, the chapter presents basic information on the use of questionnaires and interview schedules. The differences between these two forms of structured self-reports are described, with the intent of providing readers with an understanding of the situations in which one or the other techniques might be appropriate. The chapter also presents some basic concepts relating to composite self-report scales that combine multiple measures to form a single score of a particular attribute—typically a social-psychological attribute such as attitudes. Other less widely used forms of self-report (vignettes, Q-sorts, and projective techniques) are briefly described. Finally, the strengths and limitations of self-report techniques (including response set biases) are discussed. Consumers should recognize the limitations of self-report techniques as well as situations in which they are appropriate.

The next section of Chapter 11 introduces readers to procedures used to collect data by direct observation. Observational methods are often especially useful to nurse researchers since many patient outcomes are amenable to observation. Both structured and unstructured observations are described and evaluated. Finally, the issue of observational biases is discussed, and criteria for critiquing observational methods are presented.

Biophysiologic measures are discussed next. These measures have assumed greater significance to nurse researchers in the past two decades because of the growing emphasis on clinical research. Therefore, it is important for consumers to understand their applications, strengths, and limitations.

Guidelines for the critical evaluation of the various data collection approaches are presented within each major section. Separate guidelines are also presented to help consumers evaluate the procedures used to collect research data.

■ Selected Comments on the Research Examples in the Textbook

EXAMPLE 1: STRUCTURED SELF-REPORTS AND BIOPHYSIOLOGIC MEASURES

Brooks-Brunn (2000) undertook a prospective study that used quantitative data from a variety of sources to predict postoperative pulmonary complications (PPCs—the dependent variable) in women undergoing total abdominal hysterectomy. Here are a few comments on the researcher's data collection plan.

- Commendably, the researcher identified the variables she needed to include as potential predictor (independent) variables through a review of the literature. The predictors included preoperative, intraoperative, and postoperative risk factors. Unfortunately, however, Brooks-Brunn was restricted to data that were routinely available or could be obtained through interviews. She did not have the resources or authority to collect biophysiologic data that might otherwise not be required for the patient, such as pulmonary function tests for all subjects.

- Brooks-Brunn capitalized on the wealth of data available to her, however. Self-report data were collected preoperatively through in-person interviews by trained research assistants . These interviews gathered information about age, smoking history, overall health, and so on. Data from various biophysiologic measures were obtained for intraoperative and postoperative risk factors and also for the dependent variable.

- The author presented her risk factors in a succinct table so that readers could see at a glance what the independent variables were.

- There was not, however, much detail in the text about the actual measures. For example, there is no information about how "smoking history" was operationalized. As another example, there was no information on whether obesity (as assessed through the body mass index) was based on self-reported height and weight, or actual measurements. There was also information about data that were gathered that did not appear to translate into specific measures. For example, the report indicates that the subjects were interviewed every day postoperatively, but there do not appear to be any corresponding variables from these interviews. Constraints on length of the report could account in part for these ambiguities. (There was, however, a good description of how the dependent variable was operationalized.)

- The report did make clear that the researcher took great care in ensuring high-quality data, both in terms of the training of the data collectors and efforts to evaluate agreement among the data collectors about the data values. Also, Brooks-Brunn safeguarded against data collection biases of PPC predictors by not divulging subjects' PPC status to those collecting the data.

- The high degree of structure of the data collection measures seems appropriate, given the nature of the research question. However, a few open-ended questions regarding the experiences of subjects with a PPC might have enriched the study.

EXAMPLE 2: UNSTRUCTURED SELF-REPORT AND OBSERVATION

Vivian and Wilcox (2000) used various forms of unstructured data in their study of nurse-patient communication relating to compliance. Here are some comments on their methods of data collection.

- Vivian and Wilcox nicely integrated several types of data collection methods. These methods varied in terms of basic approach (self-report and observation), self-report method (personal interviews and telephone interviews), focus (from general and nonspecific during Phase I observations to more focused in Phase II interviews), setting (nurses from two home care agencies, with data collection in 25 patient homes), and type of study participants (nurses, their patients, and family members).

- The researchers used data collection methods that were well suited to their desire to understand patient compliance and the role that nurses play in encouraging and monitoring it. The researchers were able to both observe nurse-patient interaction directly and get indirect confirmatory information through interviews with the key actors. In this fashion, they were able to develop a comprehensive understanding of the phenomenon within this specific context.

- The degree of structure in their study was consistent with the study purpose. Moreover, this study exemplifies one of the advantages of a flexible data collection plan. The researchers began by making direct observations. Subsequent questioning was then developed, in part, on the basis of those observations.

- The researchers made the decision to not tape record any of the observational or interview sessions, feeling that tape recorders might have been overly obtrusive. It cannot be determined whether this decision was sound, but it must be noted that it is quite difficult to take comprehensive notes while at the same time attending to what is transpiring in the research situation. Moreover, even without tape recorders, it cannot be assumed that there was no reactivity. It might have been preferable for the researchers to make multiple observations of each patient—although that clearly would have added to the cost of doing the research.

- The researchers described their Phase I activities as "participant observation," but nothing in the description of the study confirms that the observers actually participated in the home care sessions.

■ Answers to Selected Study-Guide Questions

A.1.   1. b   2. a   3. c   4. c   5. d
       6. a   7. a   8. c   9. d   10. a

A.2.   1. c   2. b   3. a   4. a   5. c
       6. b   7. b   8. a   9. c   10. a

A.3.   1. a, c 2. a, b   3. b, c   4. c   5. b
       6. b   7. a, b, c 8. a, b   9. a, b, c 10. a

B.1.   Structure, quantifiability, researcher obtrusiveness, objectivity
   2. Historical research   3. Secondary analysis   4. Topic guide
   5. Focus group   6. Life histories   7. Closed-ended
      interview   (fixed-alternative)
   8. Open-ended   9. Closed-ended (fixed alternative)
   10. Scale   11. Declarative   12. Reversed
   13. Bipolar adjectives   14. Random   15. Extreme response
                                                           set
   16. Response set biases 17. Vignettes   18. Behavior
   19. Reactivity   20. Participant observation
   21. Single, multiple,   22. Logs, field notes
       mobile
   23. Category system   24. In vivo   25. In vitro

C.4.   Y = 11; Z = 26
C.5.   A = Acquiescence B = None C = Extreme response set   D = Nay-
       sayers' bias

D.2.   Leidig used a questionnaire in her study of adolescent drug use patterns, an efficient method of collecting data from a large sample of respondents who were geographically dispersed in twenty-five different communities. The time and expense required to interview 3,568 students would have been extremely high. There are other advantages to the use of questionnaires in this particular study. Given that the investigation concerned drug-use habits, a questionnaire that gave total anonymity probably enhanced the truthfulness of student responses. It is easier to admit to socially unacceptable behavior when one believes that no one will be able to learn your identity.

One of the chief disadvantages of questionnaires is that response rates tend to be low, resulting in the possibility of a biased sample. Leidig's method of distribution probably resulted in a fairly high response rate at a very low cost. Nonrespondents were probably primarily students not in school on the day the questionnaires were administered. Although absenteeism is undoubtedly not a random phenomenon, the bias resulting from such nonresponse may be modest. To be on the safe side, Leidig would have done well to try to administer the questionnaire to a subsample of absent students to determine the direction on any biases (if any). A more serious problem, however, is that Leidig's population appears to be defined as "urban adolescents." Since she distributed the questionnaires through the school system, adolescents who had dropped out of high school could not possibly have been included in the sample. This is an especially serious problem because high-school dropouts are probably at substantially greater risk of using drugs than are high-school students. Leidig should stipulate that her target population is urban high-school students.

Another reason for using an interview rather than a questionnaire is that one can typically get more detailed information in an interview through open-ended questions. In this study, the researcher focused primarily on descriptive information, which can easily be obtained by means of closed-ended questions. Leidig's use of primarily closed-ended questions seems appropriate in terms of her method of data collection because many students would not want to take the time to write out long essays in response to open-ended questions. However, it must be acknowledged that many interesting pieces of information about adolescent drug use would not be obtainable through a self-administered questionnaire. For example, the study would probably not shed much light on how the students started taking drugs, how they felt about their drug use, what (if anything) they had done to curtail their use, and so on.

Another risk that Leidig ran by using a questionnaire was that some students might have had reading problems; reading levels clearly are not a problem in an interview. Assuming that the researcher took care in using simple, clear questions and a well-formatted questionnaire, the use of a questionnaire in this study is probably still defensible, particularly given the other advantages of this method of data collection. One of the ways in which Leidig could have checked on the appropriateness of the questionnaire's reading level was through adequate pretesting. Her use of ten college freshmen in the pretest was not justifiable. The ability of these ten students to comprehend the questions would tell the researcher nothing about the ability of a ninth-grade student who had repeated two grades to understand the questions and how to answer them. Leidig should have administered the pretest to at least twenty to twenty-five high-school students, making sure that the pretest sample included students with low reading skills.

In summary, Leidig's distribution of questionnaires to high-school students was defensible, assuming the target population is more narrowly defined and assuming the focus is primarily on drug use incidence. In this study, interviews would have been more problematic because the sample would likely have been smaller and candor might have been lower because responses would not be anonymous. The use of self-reports was also justifiable—no other method, in fact, seems appropriate. Leidig's biggest data collection error was inadequate pretesting of the questionnaire.

D.4.   Sacks and Carter collected data on parents' experiences in caring for their dying children through in-depth interviews and observations. By using an observational approach, the researchers were able to directly see the parents' care-giving behaviors, rather than relying on their reports about their own behavior.

By using an unstructured approach, Sacks and Carter could explore the full range of the care-taking experience—not only what was being done, but also what was being said, what was *not* being done, and what was being expressed nonverbally (e.g., through body language, etc.). In other words, an unstructured approach gave the researchers the opportunity to look at the experience holistically.

Although the observation was unstructured, the approach cannot be described as participant observation. That is, the researchers did not actually care for the sick children, or engage in any other parenting behavior.

Clearly, the parents knew of the researchers' presence and knew of the purpose of the observations. It is therefore possible that reactivity was a problem—that is, that the parents' care-giving behaviors were altered because of the known presence of the researcher. However, it is commendable that the researchers made ten observations of each family over a two-month period. Undoubtedly, the reactivity problem would diminish over time as family members became more accustomed to having the researchers there. It is unlikely, though, that reactivity would disappear completely.

D.6.   Meany collected data on children's snacking behaviors by observing these behaviors in a structured setting. Because the focus of the research was on the children's selection of snacks, direct observation was a reasonable approach. Other alternatives might have been interviews with the children, interviews or questionnaires with parents, or some projective technique with the children (e.g., role playing, sentence completion). Each of these methods has problems of its own. In the case of self-reports, deliberate or unconscious distortions might have biased the results. Parents might especially tend to underreport the consumption of "junk foods" in order not to seem deficient as parents. Projective techniques might well have been used as a *supplement* to the direct observation. The use of observation alone has some limitations because Meany had no way of knowing how typical the children's snacking behavior was in the structured setting relative to, say, after-school or before-bedtime snacking.

The description suggests that no concealment was used in observing the students' choice of snacks. The method used could have created a reactivity problem. After all, school nurses are not normally present in the classroom during snack breaks. Reactivity might have been especially problematic in the experimental groups because these children would have been alert to the types of snacks the nurse would want them to choose. A better procedure might have been to have a listing of all snack foods available for selection (together with their nutritional ratings) and then to observe items *not* selected by the students after the fact. In this fashion, it would still have been possible to derive average nutritional ratings of selected food items. Reactivity would still have been a potential problem because of the presence of teachers, but reactivity would probably have been minimal. On the other hand, this approach would have required some procedure to determine that selected snacks were actually consumed—and it would have made it impossible to consider individual-level data (e.g., gender differences in program effects).

Meany elected to use a structured method of generating the behaviors to be observed (i.e., she intervened by creating snack breaks) and a structured method of recording observations. The data were easily quantified using the nutritional ratings of selected snacks. A less structured approach might have yielded more information on what the children normally eat as snacks (i.e., out of a school context), but how could observers have gained access to the students except in such a structured setting? Given the nature of the research question, the degree of structure of the observation seems justified.

Meany used event sampling to gather her data. She observed the children during several specific events, the snack break sessions. Time sampling would not have been appropriate because snacking occurred only once a week.

In summary, Meany's method of data collection was basically sound. It could have been improved if the reactivity problem had been handled better. Use of an additional method of collecting information on snacking at other times and places would also have been advisable.

D.8.   Lebowitz chose a biophysiologic measure—hematocrit readings—to evaluate the effectiveness of her nutritional intervention with pregnant women. This choice was a good one for several reasons. First, as mentioned in the text, biophysiologic measures such as this one are objective, not open to deliberate falsification because of the subject's desire to look good, and relatively sensitive indicators of subject status. Because of the investigator's interest in analyzing *change* over the course of the intervention, the chosen measure was well suited in that it could not be influenced by a testing effect (*i.e.,* the administration of the hematocrit test at the 36-week measurement was completely independent of the influence of the previous measurement). The measures were unobtrusive in the sense that the subjects were not aware that the blood tests were being used to test Lebowitz's research hypothesis that the intervention would decrease anemia (although not unobtrusive to the subjects in a general sense). Presumably, the use of hematocrit test results was also cost-effective.

On the other hand, the use of the hematocrit readings alone yielded little information about how (if at all) the intervention could be improved. The results suggested that the intervention did not have the desired effects; but this finding could reflect, for example, too small a sample or inadequate length of time between changes in nutritional habits and the final measurements. Additional data should probably have been collected to provide greater insights into the findings. In particular, Lebowitz would have been wise to collect supplementary self-report data regarding the women's nutritional practices and attitudes. Observational data would also be desirable (*e.g.,* to see what types of food the subjects ate) and could perhaps have been obtained in a structured or staged setting but would be difficult to obtain on a day-to-day basis. Such measures would not necessarily be *preferred* to physiologic measures because of the issues raised in the paragraph above, but they would have greatly enhanced Lebowitz's study if used as a supplement.

■ Test Questions and Answers

MULTIPLE CHOICE

1. Which of the following types of research does *not* use existing data?
   a. Historical research
   b. Secondary analysis
   *c. Survey research
   d. Record-based research

2. Among which of the following dimensions do self-report methods vary?
   a. Structure
   b. Quantifiability
   c. Objectivity
   *d. All of the above

3. Which of the following data collection approaches does not belong with the others?
   *a. Questionnaire
   b. Focused interview
   c. Life history
   d. Focus group interview

4. A major advantage of fixed alternative questions is that they:
   a. Are easy to construct
   *b. Are analyzed in a straightforward manner
   c. Encourage in-depth responses
   d. All of the above

5. A major purpose of a pretest of an instrument is to:
   *a. Detect inadequacies in an interview schedule or questionnaire
   b. Obtain some preliminary results on the research problem
   c. Assess the adequacy of the research design
   d. Evaluate whether an unstructured approach would be more suitable

6. Interviews are generally preferable to questionnaires because:
   - a. They are less expensive
   - b. They are easier to analyze
   - *c. The quality of the data tends to be higher
   - d. There is less opportunity for bias

7. Questionnaires have the advantage of:
   - *a. Offering the possibility of anonymity
   - b. Having high response rates
   - c. Eliminating response set biases
   - d. Being suitable for all types of respondents

8. On a five-point Likert scale, a person who neither agreed nor disagreed with the statement would be scored as:
   - a. 0
   - b. 1
   - *c. 3
   - d. 5

9. On a 20-item Likert scale with five response categories, the range of possible scores is:
   - a. 0 to 100
   - b. 20 to 80
   - *c. 20 to 100
   - d. 0 to 50.

10. A semantic differential scale consists of:
    - a. A series of declarative statements along an agree-disagree continuum
    - b. A number of test items on semantics
    - c. Items that measure facts rather than attitudes
    - *d. Sets of bipolar adjectives arranged along a continuum of degree of feeling about a concept

11. A method used to measure subjective experiences such as pain and fatigue is:
    - a. Q-sorts
    - b. Vignettes
    - *c. Visual analog scales
    - d. Projective techniques

12. The social desirability response set is least likely to be a problem on scales incorporated into which of the following?
    - *a. Mailed questionnaire
    - b. Face-to-face interview
    - c. Telephone interview
    - d. All of the above are equivalent

13. The technique that is least susceptible to response-set bias is:
    - a. Interviews
    - b. Q-sorts
    - c. Questionnaires
    - *d. Projective measures

14. Vignettes can easily be incorporated into:
    - a. Focus group interviews
    - *b. Questionnaires
    - c. Observational rating scales
    - d. Projective techniques

15. When an observer is not concealed, the findings may be biased because of:
    - *a. Reactivity
    - b. Ethical problems
    - c. Lack of mobility
    - d. Acquiescence response set

16. An observer who moves around the site to observe behaviors from different locations is using:
    a. Single positioning
    *b. Multiple positioning
    c. Mobile positioning
    d. None of the above

17. Which of the following structured observational method records the degree of behavior observed along a continuum?
    a. Category system
    b. Logs
    c. Checklist
    *d. Rating scale

18. In participant observation, data are collected in the form of:
    a. Checklists
    *b. Field notes
    c. Rating scales
    d. Questionnaires

19. A sphygmomanometer yields:
    *a. An in vivo measure
    b. An in vitro measure
    c. Either an in vivo or in vitro measure
    d. None of the above

20. Which of the following is an example of an in vitro measure?
    a. Electromyogram recordings
    b. Thermistor readings
    *c. Stool cultures
    d. Renal arteriograms

TRUE/FALSE

(T) 1. When a researcher reanalyzes previously collected data, the study is often referred to as a secondary analysis.

(T) 2. Questionnaires tend to be high on structure, quantifiability, obtrusiveness, and objectivity.

(F) 3. Most nursing research studies involve data collected by structured biophysiologic measures.

(F) 4. The greater the degree of structure an interview has, the more accurate are the results.

(F) 5. Topic guides are used to collect data in unstructured observational studies.

(F) 6. Interview schedules tend to be more structured than questionnaires.

(T) 7. A major purpose of tightly structured questionnaires is to ensure comparability of responses from subjects.

(T) 8. Closed-ended questions ask participants to choose the most appropriate answer from a list of alternatives.

(F) 9. Open-ended items are more difficult to construct than closed-ended ones.

(F) 10. Interview schedules are generally more effective than questionnaires as a means of obtaining information about socially unacceptable behaviors.

(T) 11. Questionnaires should be pretested with people whose characteristics are similar to those of the eventual study participants.

(F)   12. One of the disadvantages of telephone interviews is the low response rate.

(F)   13. The most common type of scaling procedure used in attitude measurement is the semantic differential scale.

(T)   14. In scoring a Likert scale, the values of negatively worded items should be reversed.

(F)   15. Visual analog scales involve sorting cards along a specified dimension.

(T)   16. Response-set bias refers to a person's tendency to respond characteristically in a particular way, regardless of the item's content.

(F)   17. An advantage of using the Q-sort technique is its relative ease of administration.

(T)   18. One of the problems associated with projective techniques is uncertainties in the degree to which they measure the concept they purport to measure.

(F)   19. Participant observation is a structured observational method.

(T)   20. The researcher engages in activities of the group being studied in participant observation research.

(F)   21. In time sampling, the researcher selects specific integral events for observation.

(T)   22. Reactivity refers to changes in participants' behaviors due to the known presence of an observer.

(T)   23. Biophysiologic measures may be used as either independent variables or dependent variables in a study.

(F)   24. One of the greatest strengths of biophysiologic measures is their unobtrusiveness.

Evaluating Measurements and Data Quality

■ Statement of Intent

Chapter 12 is designed to assist students in evaluating data quality. Because quantitative data are collected in most nursing studies, the beginning section of the chapter introduces students to the basic principles of measurement. A major intent here is to have students recognize that quantitative measurement is neither inherent nor arbitrary and that good measuring tools have certain attributes for which the researcher is often responsible.

The subsequent section explains how measurement error can interfere with the accuracy of quantitative measurements and indicates several sources of measurement error. The concepts of reliability and validity are then covered in some detail. Both reliability and validity have multiple aspects, each of which can be assessed differently. It is important for the student to recognize, however, that for any given instrument, some ways of assessing reliability and validity are more appropriate than others. Another important point is that the quality of an instrument partially depends on its particular application.

The section describing assessments of qualitative data-gathering methods has been further expanded in this edition. Various criteria for evaluating qualitative data quality are described, and techniques for enhancing and documenting the trustworthiness of qualitative data are reviewed.

Students should be expected to realize, after reading this chapter, that qualitative and quantitative researchers are equally interested in having their data reflect reality as accurately and truthfully as possible. Even though the terminology for assessments of quantitative and qualitative data is different, the underlying concepts are similar.

■ Selected Comments on the Research Examples in the Textbook

EXAMPLE OF AN ASSESSMENT OF A STRUCTURED SCALE

Bakas and Champion (1999) developed—and undertook a psychometric evaluation of—the Bakas Caregiving Outcomes Scale (BCOS), a scale that measures life changes for family care-givers of stroke patients. Here are several comments on the researchers' activities:

- The researchers undertook a careful, multiphase project designed to ensure the highest possible quality of the BCOS. Admirably, the initial pool of 48 items for the scale was developed on the basis of theory and was subjected to a content validation by five experts. The content validation resulted in the elimination of 21 items that at least some experts did not judge to be relevant.

- The actual evaluation of the BCOS was carried out in two phases, with refinements occurring both within each phase and across the two phases as a result of information gleaned about the reliability and validity of the BCOS.

- In terms of reliability assessments, Bakas and Champion used Cronbach's alpha to estimate internal consistency reliability, the most relevant type of reliability in this instance. Test-retest reliability would not, for example, have been appropriate because the effects of care-giving could change over time.

- The internal-consistency of the twelve-item scale developed in the first phase was .90, which was quite high. In the second phase, two additional items were omitted, and reliability coefficient for the ten-item scale was .77. In this instance, however, the reliability did not drop because two items were omitted; indeed, eliminating these two items, which had very little variability, slightly increased alpha from .75 to .77. (In general, the researchers found reliability lower in the second than in the first sample, perhaps because the sample was more homogeneous.

- In both phases, the authors tested the scale's criterion and construct validity. Factor analysis and "known groups" procedures contributed to the researchers' conclusion that the BCOS was a brief and valid indicator of care-giving effects.

- It should be noted that the final ten-item scale could not be said to be content valid because content validation was done with the full initial pool of items. A further review by a panel of experts could reveal that the ten items that remained after psychometric evaluation did not comprehensively cover the construct's domain.

EXAMPLE OF AN ASSESSMENT OF QUALITATIVE DATA

Banister (1999) collected in-depth data relating to midlife women's perceptions of their changing bodies. Banister's efforts to enhance, appraise, and describe data quality are commented on below.

- Banister documented, to a far greater degree than is typical in qualitative studies, the steps she took to improve and evaluate data quality. Her report could serve as a model of the kinds of information consumers should look for and expect in a qualitative study.

- Banister used many of the techniques suggested by Lincoln and Guba. Method triangulation was one approach used to converge on the truth: The data were gathered by both individual interviews and focus-group interviews. The focus group interviews both served as an additional data source and as an opportunity for member checking. (The study might, however, have profited from other types of triangulation, such as investigator triangulation. Banister appears to have done all coding and analysis of her data single-handedly.)

- In addition to having focus groups, Banister gave her informants opportunities to comment on the emerging conceptualization throughout the research process and invited them to "suggest changes where they felt that the materials did not reflect their experiences" (p. 525). In the absence of investigator triangulation, such member checks were crucial to enhancing data quality.

- Peer debriefing was also used to enhance the credibility of the data analysis and interpretations.

- Banister recognized that her own situation as a woman in midlife had the potential to both enhance the analysis because of personal insights and undermine it because subjective experiences could have clouded her analytic judgment. However, she wisely chose to document her reactions in a reflexive journal. This journal became part of the audit trail for the project.

- The transferability of the findings of the study were enhanced through the richness of the researcher's descriptions and her extensive use of verbatim excerpts.

■ Answers to Selected Study-Guide Questions

A.1.	1. a	2. c	3. b	4. c		
	5. a	6. b	7. d	8. b		
A.2.	1. a	2. c	3. b	4. d	5. a	6. b

B.1.	Attributes (characteristics)	2. Quantification	3. Rules
	4. Measurement error	5. True score	6. Stability
	7. Cronbach's alpha (coefficient alpha)	8. Interrater (interobserver) reliability	
	9. Valid	10. Face	11. Content
	12. Predictive	13. Construct	14. Psychometric evaluation

15. Credibility, transferability, dependability, confirmability
16. Prolonged engagement
17. Data triangulation   18. Member check
19. Confirmability
20. Inquiry audit

D.2.   Whann constructed a ten-item scale to measure paternal bonding in new fathers. To assess the scale's reliability, she used the split-half technique, which assesses the internal consistency of an instrument. Whann's focus on the homogeneity of the items in the scale was appropriate. It would probably make little sense to assess the scale's stability over time. Paternal bonding may well change on a daily basis, so a modest reliability coefficient between two administrations of the scale would not necessarily reflect unreliability, but rather true change in the attribute being measured. The equivalence aspect of reliability also is not relevant here. Although Whann did well to focus on internal consistency, she would have obtained more accurate reliability coefficients using Cronbach's alpha method. However, the split-half technique is easier to compute and is acceptable.

Whann's computations indicate that the reliability of the scale could (and should) be improved. With a reliability coefficient of .62, there is considerable measurement error. The easiest way to improve the reliability of this scale would be to add more items.

Two methods were used to evaluate the scale's validity. The content validity approach is a useful procedure to assess the comprehensiveness of the scale's questions but is not *in itself* an adequate means of ensuring the scale's validity. In this case, Whann would have benefited by obtaining information regarding the scale's content validity from more than two people.

Whann's second approach is also problematic. She used criterion-related validity, with nurses' ratings used as the criterion against which the fathers' scale scores were compared. One major problem here is that the validity of the nurses' ratings is questionable. The most defensible aspect of validity on which to focus in this case is construct validity. The known-groups technique might have been used by a comparison of scores of, for example, new fathers with fathers of 6-month-old infants (one would expect paternal bonding to be higher in the latter group).

The validity coefficient tells us very little. First, there is an upper ceiling on the validity coefficient because of the unreliability of the scale. Second, a low validity coefficient could also reflect the low validity of the nurses' ratings. Whann should add items to her scale, readminister the longer scale to a new sample, and then use a construct validation approach in estimating the scale's validity.

■ Test Questions and Answers

MULTIPLE CHOICE

1. The difference between a true score and an obtained score is referred to as:
   - a. Internal inconsistency
   - b. Equivalence
   - c. Split-half
   - *d. Error of measurement

2. One source of measurement error in social-psychological scales is:
   - *a. Response-set bias
   - b. Inefficiency
   - c. Heterogeneity
   - d. Homogeneity

3. Cronbach's alpha is used to determine which of the following instrument attributes?
   - *a. Internal consistency
   - b. Stability
   - c. Criterion validity
   - d. Construct validity

4. The situation in which interobserver reliability would be appropriate is:
   - a. Assessing the stability of a health-promoting activity scale administered on two occasions, one month apart
   - b. Determining whether items on a scale of functional ability are internally consistent
   - *c. Determining whether there is agreement between two people rating the intensity of activity of psychiatric patients
   - d. Assessing whether an observer's rating of frustration can predict nursing home residents' self-reported satisfaction with care

5. The type of validity that employs primarily judgmental rather than empirical procedures in its assessment is:
   - *a. Content
   - b. Concurrent
   - c. Predictive
   - d. Construct

6. Suppose a researcher were interested in assessing the adequacy of an instrument to measure the theoretical conceptualization of hopefulness. The type of validation procedure would most probably be:
   - a. Content
   - b. Concurrent
   - c. Predictive
   - *d. Construct

7. Which of the following terms does not belong with the other three?
   - *a. Face validity
   - b. Criterion-related validity
   - c. Predictive validity
   - d. Concurrent validity

8. Response-set biases generally lower a scale's:
   - *a. Reliability
   - b. Face validity
   - c. Errors of measurement
   - d. Transferability

9. Which of the following terms does not belong with the others?
   - a. Known-groups technique
   - *b. Audit trail
   - c. Factor analysis
   - d. Theory-based predictions

10. If both interviews and observations were used to collect data on a single construct in one study, this would be referred to as:
    - a. Data triangulation
    - b. Investigator triangulation
    - c. Theory triangulation
    - *d. Method triangulation

11. If a researcher studying family response to adolescent suicide interviewed parents and siblings independently, the method would be referred to as:
    - *a. Data triangulation
    - b. Investigator triangulation
    - c. Theory triangulation
    - d. Method triangulation

12. A member check involves reviewing data with:
    - a. An external auditor
    - b. A peer of the researcher
    - *c. A study participant
    - d. A research assistant

13. The criterion that refers to the neutrality of qualitative data is:
    - a. Credibility
    - b. Transferability
    - c. Dependability
    - *d. Confirmability

14. The use of prolonged engagement in the collection of qualitative data enhances which of the following?
    - *a. Credibility of the data
    - b. Transferability of the data
    - c. Dependability of the data
    - d. Confirmability of the data

15. An overall assessment of the adequacy of a structured self-report or observational instrument is referred to as a(n):
    - a. Triangulation
    - *b. Psychometric evaluation
    - c. Construct validation
    - d. Inquiry audit

TRUE/FALSE

(T)   1. *Measurement* may be defined as the assignment of numbers to characteristics of objects according to specified rules.

(T)   2. A good measurement tool results in a quantitative score for a single attribute of the object being measured.

(T)   3. A major purpose of measurement is to differentiate between those who possess varying amounts of the trait being studied.

(F)   4. Reliability refers to the extent to which an instrument measures the concept that the researcher thinks is being measured.

(T)   5. A reliable measure is one that minimizes the error component of an obtained score.

(F)   6. Comparing the odd-numbered and even-numbered responses of a person on a test is an example of test-retest reliability.

(T)   7. A heterogeneous sample generally produces a higher reliability coefficient than a more homogeneous sample.

(F)   8. Reliability is an inherent property of a measuring tool.

(T)   9. An instrument that is reliable for one group may not be reliable for another group.

(F)   10. Projective methods usually have a lot of face validity.

(T)   11. An achievement test that is high on content validity can nevertheless yield scores with considerable measurement error.

(F)   12. An instrument can be valid even when it is not reliable.

(F)   13. Conceptually, methods of assessing the quality of quantitative
and qualitative measures are totally distinct.

(T)   14. Persistent observation concerns the salience of data being gathered and contributes to data credibility.

(T)   15. Data triangulation involves collecting similar information on
the topics of interest from multiple sources.

(F)   16. An inquiry audit is usually performed by members of the research team.

(T)   17. Data credibility can be enhanced by a search for disconfirming
evidence.

(T)   18. Dependability of qualitative data is to the stability/reliability of
a quantitative measure what confirmability (qualitative) is to
equivalence/reliability (quantitative).

(F)   19. The concept of transferability concerns whether the researcher
gathered data in more that two sites.

(F)   20. Evidence of the trustworthiness of qualitative data is routinely
provided in research reports.

PART V

Analysis of Research Data

Analyzing Quantitative Data

■ Statement of Intent

Chapter 13 introduces students to some basic principles of quantitative analysis. The chapter covers materials that are typically included in a full-year course of statistics, but the emphasis throughout is not on computation or on understanding fundamental principles of probability. Rather, the focus is on helping consumers of nursing research studies understand how and why certain statistical procedures are used and on helping them comprehend and interpret statistics reported in research reports.

The chapter begins with a description of the four levels of measurement, followed by a discussion of elementary descriptive statistics. The chapter covers the three basic types of univariate descriptive statistics (description of the shape of a distribution, central tendency, and variability) and methods of bivariate statistics.

The next major section discusses the principles underlying tests of statistical significance. A major aim is to show students *why* inferential statistics are needed to draw conclusions about research data. As in the previous section, the discussion focuses not on calculations but rather on the logic, use, and interpretation of various statistics. In fact, in this edition *all* computations, formulas, and Greek symbols have been omitted. The bivariate tests described in the chapter include *t*-tests, analysis of variance, chi-squared tests, and product-moment correlation coefficients.

The chapter also presents some preliminary information about multivariate statistical procedures. Increasing numbers of nurse researchers are using sophisticated multivariate statistical procedures to analyze their data, and students are likely to be faced with studies in which such a procedure was used. Chapter 13 tries to familiarize readers with some of these procedures and illustrates how and when they are used. The procedures include multiple regression and analysis of covariance, with brief mention of factor analysis, discriminant function analysis, multivariate ANOVA, logistic regression, and causal modeling.

The chapter concludes with some tips on how to read and evaluate the results section of a quantitative research report.

■ Comments on the Actual Research Examples in the Textbook

EXAMPLE OF BIVARIATE INFERENTIAL STATISTICS

Lattavo and her colleagues (1995) conducted an interesting study designed to compare core pulmonary artery temperature measures with other types of temperature measures. Here are a few comments about their study.

- The researchers first used Pearson product-moment correlation coefficients to examine the direction and intensity of relationship between core PA and all other temperature measurements. The temperatures were all interval-level measures, and so it was appropriate to compute correlation coefficients.

- The findings revealed that all correlations were moderately high and significantly different from zero—that is, there likely is a true relationship between the temperature measures and not just a relationship that happened by chance in this particular sample. However, the correlation coefficients were not as substantial as might be considered ideal if one measure were being used as a substitute for the other. For example, the correlation between axillary temperature and core PA temperature was only .68, meaning that less than half of the variance in these two measures is shared ($r^2 = .46$).

- The researcher established a criterion of .80 as the amount of shared variance needed to conclude that alternative measures were reliable substitutes for core PA temperature measures. This is a fairly arbitrary criterion, but it is nevertheless a reasonable one. Moreover, the researchers substantiated their conclusions by performing paired t-tests.

- The use of paired rather than independent groups t-tests was appropriate, since the measures were from the same subjects. In these t-tests, the dependent variable was the interval-level temperature measure and the independent variable was type of measurement (e.g., core PA versus tympanic). Strictly speaking, however, the use of a series of paired t-tests was not appropriate: A repeated measures ANOVA would have been preferable since there were five separate temperature measurements. Multiple t-tests increase the risk of a Type I error. However, the t-tests were fairly consistent in indicating that core PA temperature measures were significantly different from other types of temperature measures. It seems highly likely that the researchers came to the correct conclusion based on their analysis.

- Although studies that use bivariate statistics can often be strengthened through the use of multivariate procedures, it is not clear in this study what could have been gained by using multivariate statistics. For example, ANCOVA might have been used to control extraneous variables, but with subjects serving as their own controls, all background characteristics were already controlled through the research design.

EXAMPLE OF MULTIVARIATE STATISTICAL ANALYSIS

Johnson and her co-researchers (1999) evaluated a nurse-delivered smoking cessation intervention for cardiac patients. The following comments focus mainly on their statistical analyses.

- The researchers did an excellent job with their statistical analyses and with presenting pertinent information in their report. They presented descriptive as well as inferential statistical information. The inferential statistics were used to test two formally stated directional hypotheses.

- Descriptive demographic statistics were presented in Table I, which showed group means and standard deviations for interval- and ratio-level data (e.g., age, stress scale scores) and percentages for nominal-level variables (e.g., sex, marital status). Note that some of the nominal variables were ones that *could* have been measured on a higher scale (e.g., income level at or below $40,000, rather than the actual dollar amount.) Although this table presents a wealth of information, one minor shortcoming is that the table does not specifically note that the entries are means with SDs in parentheses for interval and ratio variables.

- Further descriptive information relating to the baseline smoking characteristics of subjects in the two groups is presented in Table II. This table shows means but not SDs.

- In recognition of the fact that the design for this study was quasi-experimental, the researchers wisely collected and displayed information about preintervention group differences. They appropriately used *t*-tests and chi-squared tests to compare the two groups with respect to pre-treatment means and proportions, respectively. (The final entry under the column "Statistics" in Table II should have been a chi-squared value rather than a *t*-test value; this was likely a typographical rather than an analytic error.) These analyses, designed to shed light on the study's internal validity, revealed that the two groups were mostly similar in terms of background characteristics, except that subjects in the experimental group had significantly higher incomes, were less likely to have undergone cardiac surgery, and had higher mean scores on a social self-efficacy scale.

- This study is a good example of the importance of controlling preintervention characteristics analytically, especially when the design is not experimental. The bivariate test of the central hypothesis (which appropriately used the chi-squared test because both the independent and dependent variables were nominal-level) resulted in nonsignificant group differences, suggesting that the smoking cessation intervention had not been effective in reducing smoking. However, in the multivariate analyses (which again used an appropriate test, logistic regression), baseline characteristics were controlled. In contrast to the bivariate analysis, the multivariate analysis indicated that patients in the experimental group were significantly less likely to have resumed smoking than those in the control group. Similarly, post-intervention group differences in self-efficacy were not significant, even after controlling baseline self-efficacy scores through ANCOVA. However, when more control variables were included in the multiple regression analysis the group differences were significant. (It would appear that multiple regression analysis was used in the latter analyses rather than ANCOVA to take advantage of the "stepwise" feature of multiple regression; students should be aware, however, that ANCOVA could also have been and would have yielded the same results.)

■ Answers to Selected Study-Guide Exercises

A.1. 1.d 2.a 3.d 4.b 5.c 6.a
      7.b 8.d 9.c 10.b 11.b 12.a

A.2. 1.b 2.a 3.c 4.d 5.b
      6.b 7.a 8.a 9.c 10.a

A.3. 1.b 2.a 3.d 4.b 5.c
      6.a 7.a 8.a 9.d 10.a

B.1. Enumeration (count) 2. Ordinal 3. Zero

4. Equal distances 5. Parameter 6. Frequency distribution

7. Frequency polygons 8. Symmetric 9. Negatively

10. Unimodal 11. Normal distribution (bell-shaped curve)

12. Central tendency 13. Variability 14. Homogeneous

15. Standard deviation 16. Bivariate statistics 17. Negative (inverse)

18. Pearson's r (product—moment correlation coefficient)

19. Inferential statistics 20. Normal 21. Type I

22. Parametric 23. Levels of significance 24. Type II

25. F-ratio 26. Chi-squared test 27. Multiple regression

28. R 29. .00, 1.00 30. Analysis of covariance

31. Covariate 32. Factor analysis

33. Discriminant function analysis, logistic regression 34. Logistic regressio

35. Path analysis, LISREL (linear structual relations analysis)

C.3. Unimodal, fairly symmetric

C.4. Mean: 81.8; Median: 83; Mode: 84

C.7. a. Chi-squared b. t-test c. Pearson's r d. ANOVA

C.9. a. Discriminant function analysis or logistic regression
      b. ANCOVA   c. MANOVA   d. Multiple regression

D.2.   The following is a list of all the variables in Mouzon's study and the level of measurement for each:

absence or presence of sleep problems	nominal
amount of anesthesia	ordinal
time spent in labor	ratio
type of delivery	nominal
birth weight	ratio
Apgar score	ordinal

   The six variables in the research covered three of the four levels of measurement (Apgar scores could be categorized as interval-level variables, but are probably more accurately classified as ordinal). Most of the variables were measured on the highest possible scale, but in two instances, a higher level was possible. The first was the dependent variable, sleep-disturbance problems. An infant could be rated in terms of the degree of sleeping problems; such ratings would yield at least ordinal and perhaps interval data. Alternatively, one could use a more objective measure of sleeping behavior, such as the number of consecutive hours of sleep per night, the number of nocturnal sleep interruptions, or the number of changes from sleep to wake states per day. All these would yield ratio-level data.
   The second variable that could be measured on a higher level is the amount of anesthesia used at delivery. Here, the actual amount could be measured. It would probably be worthwhile to separate different types of anesthesia administered as well. Changes such as those suggested could, in fact, alter Mouzon's findings and conclusions.

D.4.   Balmuth appropriately used a variety of quantitative descriptive statistics for the data she collected. (Some might argue that she should have collected in-depth qualitative data instead of, or in addition to, the quantitative information, given the nature of his research question.)
   Balmuth used all five major types of descriptive statistics discussed in Chapter 13 of the text, as follows:

Frequency distribution:	self-ratings of health
Central tendency:	predicted length of stay (mean and median)
Variability:	predicted length of stay (standard deviation)
Contingency table:	mobility group by self-ratings of health
Correlation:	predicted length of stay and self-ratings of health

   Balmuth's selection of statistics generally seems appropriate for the level of measurement of the variables. For example, predicted length of stay was measured on a ratio scale; means and standard deviations are suitable. Balmuth also reported a median for this variable, and, although not necessary, this information would suggest to an alert reader that the distribution is skewed.

The self-rating, in contrast, is an ordinal-level variable. Summarizing the data on this variable by means of a frequency distribution was acceptable, although the medians also could have been computed. Similarly, rather than constructing a contingency table for this variable, Balmuth could have computed medians for each of the three groups. However, Balmuth's method is acceptable—many researchers summarize ordinal data by use of percentages.

Balmuth's presentation communicated considerable information in a short amount of space. Balmuth's data consisted of 240 values organized and integrated into a concise summary. His statement suggests that his hypothesis has some support, although inferential statistics would be needed to verify this. High-mobility patients were three times as likely to rate themselves as being healthy as were low-mobility patients. Increased mobility was also associated with fewer predicted days of hospitalization. Interestingly, variability also increased as the means increased. The high-mobility group generally agreed that their length of hospital stay would be short. In the low-mobility group, however, some patients predicted fairly short stays, whereas others thought they would be there over a month. We would have had more information on this point if Balmuth had also presented the ranges for this variable for the three groups.

D.6.   Curtis had five dependent variables, all of which were measured on an interval scale. His independent variable, age, was operationalized on a nominal scale, although it could have been measured on a ratio scale using actual ages rather than age ranges. Had Curtis used actual ages, five Pearson's r statistics could have been computed to summarize the magnitude of the relationship between age and the five test scores.

One of the difficulties of using correlational procedures, however, is that these statistics can only describe and test linear relationships (wherein the values are in a straight ascending or descending order). In the present example, the relationship between age and test scores is reasonably, but not completely, linear. For the salty test, for example, test scores decline as age increases; for the sweet test, however, the 51- to 60-year-old group has the highest scores. ANOVA procedures, which were used in this case, have the advantage of communicating a lot of information about trends in the data. The researcher could have computed a correlational statistic (preferably Pearson's r with actual age data) in addition to the ANOVA.

The table shows that there were 3 and 76 degrees of freedom (df), which is correct (4 groups minus 1 = 3; 80 subjects minus 4 groups = 76).

The results suggest that age is only weakly related to taste acuity. Only in the case of salty substances was there a significant decline with age. All other observed differences could have been the result of chance. However, the differences *might* be real; a Type II error (rejecting a false null hypothesis) might have been committed. The F values for the bitter and overall test were fairly close to achieving statistical significance. Curtis would do well to replicate his study using a larger sample and increasing the number of substances tested.

■ Test Questions and Answers

MULTIPLE CHOICE

1. The level of measurement that classifies and ranks objects in terms of the degree to which they possess the attribute of interest is:
   a. Nominal
   *b. Ordinal
   c. Interval
   d. Ratio

2. Religious affiliation is measured on the:
   *a. Nominal scale
   b. Ordinal scale
   c. Interval scale
   d. Ratio scale

3. Which of the two variables—temperature in Fahrenheit degrees or weight in kilograms—uses a higher level of measurement?
   a. Temperature in Fahrenheit degrees
   *b. Weight in kilograms
   c. Both are the same
   d. Insufficient information to make a determination

4. A record of the fluid intake, in ounces, of a postsurgical patient is an example of which level of measurement?
   a. Nominal
   b. Ordinal
   c. Interval
   *d. Ratio

5. Which level of measurement permits the researcher to add, subtract, multiply, and divide?
   a. Nominal
   b. Ordinal
   c. Interval
   *d. Ratio

6. It is not meaningful to calculate the mean with data from which of the following?
   a. Nominal measures
   b. Ordinal measures
   *c. Nominal and ordinal measures
   d. None of the above

7. Degrees such as associate's, bachelor's, master's, and doctorate correspond to measures on which of the following scales?
   a. Nominal
   *b. Ordinal
   c. Interval
   d. Ratio

8. If the bulk of scores from a test occurred at the upper end of the distribution, the distribution could be described as:
   a. Normal
   b. Bimodal
   c. Positively skewed
   *d. Negatively skewed

9. A group of 100 students took a test. The mean was 85, the standard deviation was 5, and the scores were normally distributed. About how many scores fell between 80 and 90?
   a. 40
   *b. 68
   c. 95
   d. Impossible to determine

10. A parameter is a characteristic of:
    *a. A population
    b. A frequency distribution
    c. A sample
    d. A normal curve

11. The mode is an index of:
    a. Bivariate relationships
    *b. Central tendency
    c. Skewness
    d. Variability

12. The measure of variability that takes into account all score values is the:
    a. Range
    b. Median
    c. Mean
    *d. Standard deviation

13. The measure of central tendency that is most stable is the:
    a. Mode
    b. Median
    *c. Mean
    d. They are all equivalent

14. If a variable were measured on a nominal scale, the most appropriate measure of central tendency would be the:
    *a. Mode
    b. Median
    c. Mean
    d. They are all equivalent

15. Which of the following is an example of a bivariate descriptive statistic?
    a. Frequency distribution
    b. Mean
    c. Range
    *d. Correlation coefficient

16. One of the characteristics of a normal distribution is that:
    a. It is bimodal
    *b. 68% of the values are within one standard deviation above and below the mean
    c. The values are positively skewed
    d. The mean is 100

17. The symbol $\bar{X}$ represents:
    a. The standard deviation
    *b. The mean
    c. The total sample size
    d. An individual score

18. The use of inferential statistics permits the researcher to:
    *a. Draw conclusions about a population based on information gathered from a sample
    b. Describe information obtained from empirical observation
    c. Interpret descriptive statistics
    d. None of the above

19. The standard deviation of a sampling distribution is called a:
    a. Sampling error
    *b. Standard error
    c. Variance
    d. Parameter

20. The steps involved in using test statistics include all the following *except:*
    a. Determining the appropriate statistic to be used
    b. Selecting a level of significance
    c. Determining the degrees of freedom
    *d. Calculating the theoretical distribution for the test statistic

21. A major factor that affects the standard error of the mean is the:
    a. Value of the score range
    b. Sampling distribution
    *c. Sample size
    d. Value of the mean

22. For which of the following levels of significance is the risk of making a *Type II* error greatest?
    a. .10
    b. .05
    c. .01
    *d. .001

23. If a researcher calculated a *t*-statistic to be −2.2 and the tabled *t* value (for a *df* of 60 and level of significance of .05) is 2.0, the researcher would:
    a. Conclude that an error in calculation had been made
    b. Accept the null hypothesis
    *c. Reject the null hypothesis
    d. Use a different level of significance

24. A statistical procedure that is used to determine whether a significant difference exists between any number of group means on a dependent variable measured on an interval scale is the:
    a. *t*-test
    *b. ANOVA
    c. Pearson's *r*
    d. Chi-squared test

25. How many null hypotheses would there be for a study with 40 subjects, using a two-way ANOVA?
    a. 2
    *b. 3
    c. 5
    d. 10

26. If a researcher wanted to determine whether observed proportions differed significantly from expected proportions, the statistical test would be a(n):
    a. *t*-test
    b. Correlation coefficient
    c. Analysis of variance
    *d. Chi-squared test

27. When both the independent and dependent variables are measured on a ratio scale, the appropriate test statistic is a(n):
    a. *t*-test
    b. ANOVA
    c. Chi-squared test
    *d. Pearson's *r*

28. A researcher wanted to predict whether nursing home residents would or would not experience a fall based on ten characteristics (e.g., age, presence or absence of dementia, etc.). The analysis would involve:
    a. Multiple regression
    b. ANCOVA
    *c. Discriminant function analysis
    d. Factor analysis

29. A researcher wanted to compare men and women in terms of satisfaction with nursing care, controlling for age and severity of illness. The analysis would involve:
    a. Multiple regression
    *b. ANCOVA
    c. Discriminant function analysis
    d. Factor analysis

30. Suppose a researcher found a multiple correlation of .40 between candy intake, age, and dental caries. The amount of variability that could be accounted for in dental caries by candy intake and age is:
    a. 4%   c. 40%
    *b. 16%   d. Cannot be determined

31. The multivariate procedure that reduces a large set of data into a more compact set of measures is:
    a. MANOVA   c. Discriminant function analysis
    *b. Factor analysis   d. Multiple regression

32. In analysis of covariance, a covariate is generally:
    a. An independent variable   c. Either an independent or
    b. The dependent variable   dependent variable
                                    *d. An extraneous variable

TRUE/FALSE

(F)   1. Researchers use descriptive statistics to draw conclusions about population values.

(F)   2. The type of graph that depicts the relation between two or more variables is called a frequency polygon.

(F)   3. A descriptive index from a population is called a statistic.

(T)   4. A frequency distribution is a systematic arrangement of scores according to the number of times each occurred.

(T)   5. The three characteristics that can completely summarize a set of data are the shape of the distribution, central tendency, and variability.

(F)   6. "Age at death" is an example of a positively skewed attribute.

(F)   7. The median is affected by the value of each individual score.

(T)   8. The standard deviation is a measure that tells how spread out scores are in a distribution.

(F)   9. Two sets of data with identical means would likely have the same standard deviation.

(T)   10. The standard deviation represents the average of the deviations from the mean.

(F)   11. A +.50 correlation coefficient indicates a stronger relation than does a correlation of −.75.

(F)   12. Contingency tables are normally constructed with variables measured on the interval scale.

(F)   13. The tendency for statistical values to differ from one sample to another is known as the standard error of the mean.

(F)   14. As sample size decreases, so does the standard error of the mean.

(F)   15. A Type I error refers to the researcher's concluding that no difference exists when, in fact, a difference does exist.

(T) 16. A researcher never knows whether an error has been committed in statistical decision making.

(T) 17. A statistically significant finding means that the obtained results are not likely to have been due to chance.

(F) 18. Parametric tests make no assumptions about the shape of the distribution in the population.

(T) 19. The *t*-test can be used for both between-subjects and within-subject comparisons.

(F) 20. A researcher would test the difference between the means of three groups of students using a *t*-test for independent samples.

(T) 21. Nonparametric tests have fewer assumptions than parametric tests.

(F) 22. The chi-squared statistic may be considered to be both descriptive and inferential.

(F) 23. The square root of R tells how much variability in the dependent variable can be explained by the independent variables.

(T) 24. In a multiple regression analysis, the dependent variable is measured on an interval or ratio scale.

(T) 25. In ANCOVA, the effect of covariates on the dependent variable is first removed and then the relationship between the independent and dependent variables is evaluated.

(T) 26. Variables are not classified as independent or dependent in factor analysis.

(F) 27. MANOVA is the procedures used in causal modeling.

(T) 28. In logistic regression, the dependent variable is measured on the nominal scale.

(F) 29. In the following statement of results, the *df* stands for "direct F-ratio": $F = 5.2$, $df = 1.55$, $p < .05$.

(T) 30. In the following statement of results, the results are not statistically significant at conventional levels: ($r = .12$, $df = 33$, $p > .05$).

CHAPTER 14

Analyzing Qualitative Data

■ Statement of Intent

The purpose of Chapter 14 is to acquaint students with some of the fundamental principles of analyzing narrative data from unstructured interviews and observations, as well as from written documents such as diaries and letters. The chapter begins by discussing the aims of qualitative research and describing the challenges that qualitative data analysts face. The next section discusses four major analysis styles that range on a continuum from standardized and systematic to intuitive and interpretive.

While the results of qualitative analysis are usually easy for students to understand, it is often difficult to comprehend the *process* of the analysis—particularly because there are no firmly established rules. For this reason, the chapter devotes a disproportionate amount of time discussing the methods associated with grounded theory, about which much has been written. Some basic procedures that are typically used for analyzing qualitative data are also presented, but these are not described in detail. The important point to emphasize is that the analysis of qualitative data is an inductively driven process that typically uses an iterative approach of gleaning meaning from the data and checking that meaning back against the data and, often, against the interpretation of others, including the informants.

■ Selected Comments on the Research Examples in the Textbook

EXAMPLE OF A GROUNDED THEORY ANALYSIS

Durham's (1999) study of home management of preterm labor has both strengths and limitations. Here are a few comments regarding this study:

- Grounded theory was the appropriate qualitative design to investigate the process women go through to manage their treatment for preterm labor.
- The report described the process of data collection, coding, and data analysis in more detail than is typical. However, the description was fairly general. Durham did not offer specific examples of the steps she took (e.g., a specific memo illustrating how categories were linked), which would have clarified the research process.

- Because data collection and analysis occurred simultaneously (as is appropriate in a grounded theory study), and also because of the flexibility of grounded theory methodology, Durham used her emerging conceptualization to determine her data needs in her later interviews and in her follow-up interviews. However, from the reader's perspective, a specific example of how this actually worked would have been helpful.

- Durham took several steps to enhance the credibility of her grounded theory. For example, she verified her emerging conceptualization in follow-up interviews with six women. Furthermore, Durham had ongoing discussions with a qualitative research group (i.e., with a group of peers).

- Another strength of the study is that Durham continued to collect data until saturation occurred.

- Given Durham's interest in describing a *process,* it is noteworthy that she interviewed women at different phases of managing preterm labor. At the time of the interviews, the women had been treated for preterm labor for varying lengths of time, ranging from 1.5 to thirteen weeks. Moreover, she conducted follow-up interviews with six women, which presumably provided a longitudinal perspective.

- Regrettably, the report did not provide information about the follow-up interviews. That is, Durham did not explain the main purpose of the follow-up, why only six women were reinterviewed, how those six women were chosen, what type of information was obtained, and so on.

- Durham described in depth the three-stage process of negotiating activity restriction, with rich, enlivening excerpts from the interviews that help to give readers a stronger sense of the validity of the conclusions.

- One concern, however, is that it appears that the researcher may have begun data collection already assuming what the basic social process was for these women, namely negotiating activity restriction. In grounded theory studies, the basic social process should emerge from the data.

- It is important to note that the sample primarily comprised white, professional middle-class women who lived with a male partner. Thus, the findings may not be applicable to single women from different ethnic and socioeconomic backgrounds.

EXAMPLE OF AN ANALYSIS FROM AN ETHNOGRAPHIC STUDY

Russell's (1996) ethnographic study of care-seeking among elders in a retirement community resulted in a voluminous amount of data that needed to be analyzed. Here are a few comments regarding her qualitative analysis.

- Russell gathered a variety of data from different sources (personal interviews, observations, and a focus group interview), which enabled her to get divergent perspectives on elders' care-seeking behavior. In addition to method triangulation, Russell used a strategy of prolonged engagement (i.e., lengthy fieldwork) to enhance the credibility of her data.

- Russell collected and analyzed her data simultaneously, which gave her insights into the types of data she needed to collect to enhance her analysis.

- Like most qualitative researchers in this era, Russell used a computer to organize and manage her voluminous data.

- Russell's study is ethnographic, but it is difficult to draw conclusions about the overall analysis style. The codebook she developed could be interpreted as a template (i.e., template analysis style) or as a categorization scheme as part of an editing analysis style. Many of the ways in which Russell described her analysis suggest some methods derived from grounded theory.

- Russell's analysis suggested a two-phase care-seeking process with multiple stages in each. Her report used several excerpts from participant observation notes and interviews to illustrate and substantiate her interpretation of that process.

EXAMPLE OF AN ANALYSIS FROM A PHENOMENOLOGICAL STUDY

The following are some comments on Beck's (1998) study of mothers' experience of panic disorder during the pospartum period.

- A phenomenologic design was an appropriate choice to describe the meaning of women's experience with panic after the birth of their babies.

- In keeping with the tenets of descriptive phenomenology, the researcher bracketed her presuppositions regarding postpartum onset of panic disorder prior to data collection.

- Beck used purposive sampling to select study participants, which is consistent with a phenomenologic approach.

- Appropriately, data collection continued until repetition of themes occurred.

- All of the steps of Colaizzi's method of data analysis were described. However, a specific example of a portion of Beck's audit trail would have been helpful to further explicate the data analysis process.

- The six themes concerning the meaning of panic for new mothers were described in depth. Many powerful quotes from the mothers' interviews were included in the results section.

- The researcher addressed the trustworthiness of her findings by describing the steps she had taken to ensure their credibility and auditability.

■ Answers to Selected Study-Guide Exercises

A. 1. a   2. d   3. c   4. a   5. b   6. b

B.
1. Simultaneously
2. Comprehending, synthesizing, theorizing, recontextualizing
3. Indexing, categorizing
4. Constant comparison
5. Open coding
6. Conceptual file
7. Computer programs
8. Themes
9. Quasi-statistics
10. Selective
11. Basic social process
12. Phenomenologic
13. Detailed

D. 2.   DelSette collected data on the experiences of patients who were on precautions. A qualitative approach was appropriate for the phenomenon being studied. Because the focus of the research was on patients' perspectives, direct observation and unstructured interviewing were reasonable methods of data collection. The researcher might have used more in-depth interviewing as data collection progressed; she also might have quantified her observations to determine the frequency of occurrence of relevant behaviors and incidents.

A time sampling plan was used in the observations. Observational periods spanned days, evenings, and nights. DelSette might have chosen to randomly sample the various times at which data would be collected rather than adhering to a rigid structure. A random procedure might have reduced reactivity. That is, a random observation plan would have made it more difficult for hospital staff to plan the times of their interactions. Although reactivity would probably still have been present, it might have been reduced.

DelSette recorded her observations after each two-hour observation segment. It is not clear from the study summary what is meant by "immediately following" the observation. If other events occurred, such as driving home, it is conceivable that the researcher may have rehearsed what would be entered in the notes and unconsciously altered the observations or comments. A better plan might have been to carry a small notebook for jotting down events or statements made by patients during each observation.

The field notes consisted of observational notes, personal notes, and theoretical notes. Note taking might have been improved by including any methodological changes during the course of the study. For example, DelSette might have decided to observe the positioning of patients when comments were made to the researcher concerning frustrations.

DelSette reread the field notes at the end of each four hours of observation. She handled the concept of theoretical saturation by not recording redundant information once a category had evolved. Such an approach seems logical and appropriate. Review of the field notes at specified times and their referencing according to categorical themes appeared to indicate that sufficient evidence had been collected.

The validation procedures of the study could have been improved greatly by having another researcher read the field notes and identify categories and by checking out the interpretations that DelSette gleaned from the data with the patients. The use of these two validation methods would have improved the quality of the study. DelSette appears to have validated her observations with interview material (methodological triangulation), which, while desirable and appropriate, would have profited by being supplemented by other procedures.

The categories that emerged from the data appear to be appropriate and to reflect accurately the data that were collected. However, the categories are all in the realm of feelings, and one wonders whether the data may contain other types of categories that are in the realms of physical care, activities performed by patients, and physiologic adaptations. Without reading the entire set of field notes, it would be impossible to suggest other categories that might have emerged from the data.

■ Test Questions and Answers

MULTIPLE CHOICE

1. The analysis style that is sometimes referred to as manifest content analysis is:
   *a. Quasi-statistical style
   b. Template analysis style
   c. Editing analysis style
   d. Immersion/crystallization style

2. The researcher acts as an interpreter who reads through data and develops a categorization scheme on the basis of meaningful segments in the analysis style referred to as:
   a. Quasi-statistical style
   b. Template analysis style
   *c. Editing analysis style
   d. Immersion/crystallization style

3. Which of the following is *not* a process that plays a role in qualitative analysis:
   a. Comprehending
   *b. Attributing
   c. Synthesizing
   d. Theorizing

4. The first major step that a researcher must undertake in a qualitative analysis is:
   a. A search for major themes
   b. Entering information into files
   c. The use of quasi-statistics
   *d. Developing a system for organizing and indexing the data

5. Before the advent of computer programs for qualitative analysis, the main procedure for managing qualitative data was the development of:
   *a. Conceptual files
   b. Core categories
   c. Memos
   d. Themes

6. The process referred to as *constant comparison* involves:
    a. Comparing two researchers' interpretation of the data
    b. Comparing the researchers' interpretation of the data against study participants' interpretation
    *c. Comparing data segments against other segments for similarity and dissimilarity
    d. Comparing data from one study with data from other similar studies

7. Steps generally employed in the analysis of qualitative data include all of the following *except*:
    *a. Testing hypotheses
    b. Searching for themes
    c. Validating themes
    d. Developing a coding scheme

8. Quasi-statistics is essentially a method of:
    a. Statistical analysis
    *b. Validation
    c. Thematic generation
    d. Analytic induction

9. In a grounded theory study, the first stage of coding is referred to as:
    *a. Open coding
    b. Selective coding
    c. Substantive coding
    d. Theoretical coding

10. Selective coding begins when:
    a. Constant comparison has ended
    b. Data saturation has occurred
    c. Memos have been prepared
    *d. A core variable has been identified

TRUE/FALSE

(F) 1. One of the features of qualitative analysis is that there are a number of universal formal rules that facilitate the process.

(T) 2. The continuum of qualitative analysis styles ranges from a systematic, standardized style (quasi-statistical) to an intuitive and interpretive style (immersion/crystallization).

(T) 3. The process of *comprehending* is completed when data saturation is achieved.

(F) 4. The process of *recontextualization* involves a sifting of the data and putting pieces together.

(F) 5. Coding schemes are generally developed after the completion of a thematic analysis.

(T) 6. Like quantitative analysts, qualitative analysts may search for relationships and patterns within the data.

(T) 7. Quasi-statistics involves an accounting of the frequency with which themes are and are not supported by qualitative data.

(F) 8. The grounded theory approach is applied to qualitative data after they have been gathered in the field.

(F) 9. The grounded theory analyst documents assumptions, insights, and the conceptual scheme on memos once all the data have been analyzed.

(T)   10. The Duquesne school of phenomenology yielded several different methods of analyzing descriptive phenomenological data.

(F)   11. Both grounded theory and phenomenological analysis focus on a search for themes.

(T)   12. Some approaches to phenomenological analysis require member checking, while others eschew it.

PART VI

Critical Appraisal and Utilization of Nursing Research

CHAPTER 15

Critiquing Research Reports

■ Statement of Intent

The major purpose of Chapter 15 is to provide an overall framework for the preparation of a written research critique. The chapter emphasizes that a critique of a study does not mean an exclusive focus on its flaws but rather a balanced assessment of its strengths and weaknesses. A critique essentially involves appraising the decisions the researcher has made in terms of the research problem itself, the theoretical context, methodologic strategies, handling of ethical concerns, and the manner in which the study is described in the report.

In terms of the study methodology, the major decisions that researchers face are different for qualitative and quantitative studies. In quantitative studies, the four most important decisions that a researcher typically faces concern the research design, the specification of the population and the sampling plan, the data collection plan, and the data analysis strategy. In qualitative studies, the key methodological decisions concern setting, data sources, study participants, and data quality and data analysis. These key decisions should be critiqued with particular care by reviewers.

One final dimension with which the reviewer must be concerned is the researcher's interpretation of the findings. The chapter offers some guidelines for making sense of findings in qualitative studies and in quantitative studies in which the results support the research hypotheses, fail to support them, are contrary to them, and are mixed.

■ Answers to Selected Study-Guide Exercises

A.1.   1. b   2. c   3. b   4. d   5. b
       6. a   7. d   8. c   9. a   10. a

A.2.   1. b   2.c   3.d   4.b   5.b   6.a   7.c   8.d

B. 1. Accuracy   2. Hypotheses   3. Causation
    4. Their data   5. Important (useful)   6. Decisions
    7. Strengths, weak-   8. Substantive/theoretical
       nesses (virtues, flaws)
    9. Methodologic   10. Ethical   11. Interpretive
   12. Stylistic/presentational

▪ Test Questions and Answers

MULTIPLE CHOICE

1. The major purpose of a research critique is to assess:
   a. The adequacies of a research study
   b. The inadequacies of a research study
   *c. Both of the above
   d. Neither of the above

2. The person who critiques a published research report should strive to:
   a. Withhold overly critical comments that would discourage the researcher
   b. Be as succinct as possible
   c. Judge the merits of the study based on the researcher's background
   *d. Remain as objective as possible

3. All the following questions would be appropriate to ask in evaluating both qualitative or quantitative studies *except:*
   a. Is there a clearly articulated problem statement?
   b. Are the references cited in the literature review current and appropriate?
   *c. Are extraneous variables successfully controlled?
   d. Are clinical implications discussed?

4. Which of the following statements is true?
   a. The results of statistical tests have direct meaning.
   *b. Evaluating the credibility of a study primarily concerns an assessment of methodologic decisions.
   c. Support of a researcher's hypothesis through statistical testing offers proof of its veracity.
   d. A correlation between two variables indicates that the independent variable caused the dependent variable.

5. When a researcher makes a Type II error (concludes that no relationship between the independent and dependent variables exists when in fact it does), this could occur because of:
   a. Inadequate sample size
   b. Unreliable data collection instruments
   c. Failure to control extraneous variables
   *d. All of the above

6. When a researcher obtains significant results that are opposite to what was originally hypothesized, it is likely that this occurred because of:
   a. Inadequate sample size
   b. Unreliable data collection instruments
   c. A flawed statistical analysis
   *d. Faulty reasoning

7. A reviewer's concern about the adequacy of the researcher's control over extraneous variables would be focusing on which dimension?
   a. Substantive
   *b. Methodologic
   c. Ethical
   d. Stylistic

8. A reviewer's concern about the study's relevance to nursing would be focusing on which dimension?
   *a. Substantive
   b. Methodologic
   c. Ethical
   d. Stylistic

TRUE/FALSE

(T) 1. Most research studies have inadequacies as well as adequacies.

(T) 2. Nonsignificant results pose special interpretive problems because statistical testing is designed to disconfirm the null hypothesis.

(F) 3. Publication of a research report indicates that the project was of high scientific quality.

(F) 4. Published studies are as likely to be ones with nonsignificant results as with significant results.

(F) 5. Nonsignificant results cannot be clinically important.

(T) 6. It is easier to directly evaluate the credibility of qualitative studies than quantitative studies.

(T) 7. Flaws in the research design are a more serious limitation to the quality of a research project than are gaps in the literature review.

(F) 8. The major focus of a research critique is the evaluation of the analyses and results.

(T) 9. A question that should be asked in a critique of all research reports is, "Does the report describe the rationale for methodological decisions?"

(F) 10. Because of the in-depth nature of qualitative studies, the results are never shallow.

CHAPTER 16

Using Research Findings in Nursing Practice

■ Statement of Intent

The purpose of this chapter is to sensitize nurses and nursing students to the need for increased utilization of findings from nursing research investigations. Although research utilization is often beyond the control of individual clinical nurses, the entire nursing community has a role to play in making sure that nursing practice is evidence-based.

This chapter describes both the potential for utilizing research findings and the current status of utilization—descriptions that illuminate the current gap between knowledge production and knowledge utilization. The chapter discusses some of the barriers to research utilization and suggests some strategies for overcoming those barriers. The concluding section of the chapter discusses models for undertaking both individual and organizational utilization projects.

■ Selected Comments on the Research Example in the Textbook

Sampselle and her research team (2000) conducted an important research utilization project designed to develop an evidence-based protocol for the evaluation and treatment of urinary incontinence in women. Here are some selected comments about the project.

- The research team selected a topic of great clinical significance—and one about which a sound base of knowledge existed. Thus, the team met the first two criteria for a successful utilization project.

- Laudably, the two research reports provide a very good description of how the utilization project was conceived and what the goals were. It would appear from the description that the project had both knowledge-based and problem-based triggers. That is, an organization devoted to women's health (AWHONN) specifically sought to identify a problem for its third major utilization project that was clinically noteworthy and about which considerable research existed.

- As described in the report, the project was carefully developed by a research team—with input from a team of advisors—to include a planning, implementation, and evaluation phase. The researchers appear to have given themselves sufficient time in each phase to ensure high-quality work.

- The project had a firm foundation in the AHCPR clinical practice guidelines, which themselves were based on an extensive review of the literature. However, the research team supplemented information from the AHCPR guidelines with additional literature searches and critiques. In this fashion, the team ensured that they had state-of-the-art knowledge on which to base their protocols and forms.

- The report does not make clear the extent to which the project's implementation potential was assessed before proceeding to the next phase of the project (although such an asessment may well have occurred). The team did obtain some information about implementation potential by pilot testing the data collection instruments in four sites.

- The research team established clearly articulated criteria for selecting sites at which the protocols would be tested. A total of thirty-six sites was initially selected for the implementation—an exceptionally large representation for testing the innovation. Note, however, that participating sites volunteered to be included in the project by responding to a letter mailed to the total AWHONN membership. The report does not describe the characteristics of sites that did not volunteer. Nevertheless, the report does indicate that the thirty-six sites (including the 21 that ultimately provided data and the 15 sites that dropped out of the project) "reflects the range of ambulatory care sites in the United States" (p. 15). Moreover, the researcher documented that the 1,474 cases screened in the twenty-one participating sites included women who varied in age and ethnic background. Thus, the researchers established evidence that the results of the project were likely to be transferable to other settings.

- Another noteworthy feature of the project was that all of the site coordinators responsible for implementing the project received what appears to have been excellent training. Even the training sessions were evaluated.

- The report describes both the *process* and the *outcomes* of the utilization project. Data were gathered relating to the actual experience of implementing the protocols, which revealed both positive experiences (greater professional satisfaction, greater awareness of urinary incontinence as a problem) and negative ones (increased time pressures, billing problems).

- With respect to the evaluation of patient outcomes, the team tested six specific hypotheses. Because the project had a firm knowledge base, the hypotheses were, appropriately, directional.

- Although the evaluation design was a relatively weak pre-experimental design, it is important to note that this project was not intended to *establish* a knowledge base, but rather to examine whether the existing knowledge base would support an innovation that (a) could be implemented on a broad scale and (b) would yield results consistent with prior, more rigorous research.

- Relatedly, as a knowledge-generating research project, the project would be susceptible to criticism about the high rate of attrition for follow-up data. Of the 842 women who screened positive for urinary incontinence using the protocols, only 132 provided feedback at the four-month follow-up. However, the findings from these women were consistent with the researchers' hypotheses and with prior research, lending credibility to the findings. Moreover, the researchers documented that the 132 women had significantly greater problems with urinary incontinence than those who were not followed-up.

- The researchers concluded that more research and more outreach was needed with African American and Latina women, who had a disproportionately high rate of attrition from the project.

- Overall, the quality of work in this utilization project was outstanding.

■ Answers to Selected Study Guide Exercises

A.1. c (also d) 2. a   3. b (also a, c, d)   4. d
   5. a   6. a (also b, c, and d) 7. c (also a, b, and d)
   8. d   9. b (also d)   10. c (also b and d)

B. 1. Research   2. Gap
       utilization
    3. Conduct and Utilization of Research in Nursing (CURN)
    4. Replicated   5. Stetler
    6. Knowledge-focused, problem-focused   7. Implementation potential
    8. Transferability   9. The cost/benefit of not implementing it
   10. Evaluation

■ Test Questions and Answers

MULTIPLE CHOICE

1. If a specific nursing procedure in a hospital were modified on the basis of research findings, this would be an example of:
   a. Persuasion stage of adoption   *c. Instrumental utilization
   b. Awareness stage of adoption   d. Conceptual utilization

2. The awareness stage of adoption is similar to:
   *a. Conceptual utilization   c. Decision accretion
   b. Instrumental utilization   d. None of the above

3. Utilization projects such as the WICHE and the CURN Projects revealed that research utilization is impeded by:

   *a. The shortage of reliable, methodologically sound nursing studies with clear clinical implications

   b. The shortage of publication outlets for nurse researchers

   c. The long time lag between completion of a study and the appearance of the research report in nursing journals

   d. Lack of support for research and utilization from the federal government

4. Which of the following is *not* a major barrier to research utilization in nursing?

   a. The fact that many nurses are not academically prepared to evaluate critically nursing research studies

   b. The failure of hospitals and other organizations that employ nurses to reward nurses for research utilization

   c. The low number of replications of nursing studies that show promise for utilization

   *d. The shortage of clinically relevant nursing studies

5. Researchers can improve the prospects for utilization by doing all of the following *except:*

   a. Conducting high-quality, methodologically sound studies

   b. Disseminating results to a broad audience

   *c. Offering clinical nurses resource support for a utilization project

   d. Discussing the clinical implications of their study results in their research reports

6. Which of the following strategies for utilization is *most* amenable to adoption by nursing students and clinical nurses?

   a. Preparing integrative reviews

   b. Replicating research studies

   c. Making presentations at nursing conferences

   *d. Reading professional journals widely and critically

7. An assessment of the implementation potential of a nursing innovation includes which of the following activities?

   a. Assessment of clinical relevance

   *b. Assessment of likely costs and benefits

   c. Assessment of the study's generalizability

   d. Assessment of the scientific merit of the study

8. If a finding reported in the research literature is judged not to be clinically relevant, the next step would be to:

*a. Search for another topic in the research literature

c. Assess the transferability of the findings to a new setting

b. Evaluate the scientific merit of the studies in which similar findings were obtained

d. Determine the costs and benefits of implementing the innovation

TRUE/FALSE

(T)   1. Conceptual utilization of research involves a situation in which individuals are influenced in their thinking about an issue based on their knowledge of a study.

(F)   2. Decision accretion occurs when a nurse decides to implement the findings from a rigorous research investigation.

(F)   3. Studies have generally found that nurses have failed to utilize research findings at any point along the utilization continuum.

(T)   4. The persuasion stage of adoption refers to a situation in which consumers are aware of a research finding and believe that it should result in changes.

(F)   5. A well-known nursing research utilization project is the ANA's Project on Standards of Nursing Practice.

(T)   6. Communication problems between nurse researchers and clinical nurses is a stumbling block to utilization.

(T)   7. Replication of studies must be a critical part of efforts to increase research utilization.

(T)   8. An important aspect of assessing the implementation potential of an innovation is evaluating the transferability of the findings to a new setting.

(F)   9. Knowledge-focused triggers to utilization arise from nurses' experiential, clinical knowledge.

(F)   10. A study with scientific merit necessarily has high implementation potential.

Transparency Masters to Accompany
Essentials of NURSING RESEARCH
Methods, Appraisal and Utilization, 5th Edition

Denise F. Polit, Cheryl Tatano Beck, Bernadette P. Hungler

BOX 3-2

SUMMARY OF A FICTITIOUS STUDY FOR TRANSLATION

Purpose of the study	The potentially negative sequelae of having an abortion on the psychological adjustment of adolescents have not been adequately studied. The present study sought to determine whether alternative pregnancy resolution decisions have different long-term effects on the psychological functioning of young women.	Need for the study
Research design	Three groups of low-income pregnant teenagers attending an inner-city clinic were the <u>subjects</u> in this study: those who delivered and kept the baby; those who delivered and relinquished the baby for adoption; and those who had an abortion. There were 25 subjects in each group.	Study population
Research instruments	The study <u>instruments</u> included a self-administered <u>questionnaire</u> and a battery of psychological tests measuring depression, anxiety, and psychosomatic symptoms. The instruments were administered upon entry into the study (when the subjects first came to the clinic) and then 1 year after termination of the pregnancy.	Research sample Research design & data collection procedures
Data analysis procedure	The <u>data</u> were analyzed using <u>analysis of variance (ANOVA)</u>. The ANOVA tests indicated that the three groups did not differ significantly in terms of depression, anxiety, or psychosomatic symptoms at the initial testing. At the <u>posttest</u>, however, the abortion group had significantly higher scores on the depression scale, and these girls were significantly more likely than the two delivery groups to report severe tension headaches. There were no <u>significant</u> differences on any of the <u>dependent variables</u> for the two delivery groups.	Results
Implications	The results of this study suggest that young women who elect to have an abortion may experience a number of long-term negative consequences. It would appear that appropriate efforts should be made to follow-up abortion patients to determine their need for suitable treatment.	Interpretation

Copyright © 2001 by Lippincott Williams and Wilkins.
Instructor's Resource Manual and Testbank to Accompany Essentials of Nursing Research, fifth edition by Denise F. Polit, Cheryl Tatano Beck and Bernadette P. Hungler.

BOX 4-1 ▣

POTENTIAL BENEFITS AND COSTS OF RESEARCH TO PARTICIPANTS

Major Potential Benefits to Participants

Access to an intervention to which they otherwise may not have access

Gratification in being able to discuss their situation or problem with a nonjudgmental and friendly person

Increased knowledge about themselves or their conditions, either through opportunity for introspection and self-reflection or through direct interaction with the researcher

Escape from normal routine and excitement of being part of a study

Satisfaction that the information they provide may help others with similar problems or conditions

Direct monetary or material gains through stipends or other incentives

Major Potential Costs to Participants

Physical harm, including unanticipated side effects

Physical discomfort, fatigue, or boredom

Psychological or emotional distress resulting from self-disclosure, introspection, fear of the unknown or interacting with strangers, fear of eventual repercussions, anger or embarrassment at the type of questions being asked

Loss of privacy

Loss of time

Monetary costs (*e.g.,* for transportation, child care, or time lost from work)

Copyright © 2001 by Lippincott Williams and Wilkins.
Instructor's Resource Manual and Testbank to Accompany Essentials of Nursing Research, fifth edition by Denise F. Polit, Cheryl Tatano Beck and Bernadette P. Hungler.

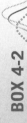

BOX 4-2

GUIDELINES FOR CRITIQUING THE ETHICAL ASPECTS OF A STUDY

1. Were the study participants subjected to any physical harm, discomfort, or psychological distress? Did the researchers take appropriate steps to remove or prevent the harm?

2. Did the benefits to participants outweigh any potential risks or actual discomfort they experienced? Did the benefits to society outweigh the costs to participants?

3. Was any type of coercion or undue influence used in recruiting participants? Were vulnerable subjects used?

4. Were participants deceived in any way? Were they fully aware of participating in a study, and did they understand the purpose of the research? Were appropriate consent procedures implemented?

5. Were appropriate steps taken to safeguard the privacy of participants?

6. Was the research approved and monitored by an Institutional Review Board or other similar ethics review committee?

Copyright © 2001 by Lippincott Williams and Wilkins.
Instructor's Resource Manual and Testbank to Accompany Essentials of Nursing Research, fifth edition by Denise F. Polit, Cheryl Tatano Beck and Bernadette P. Hungler.

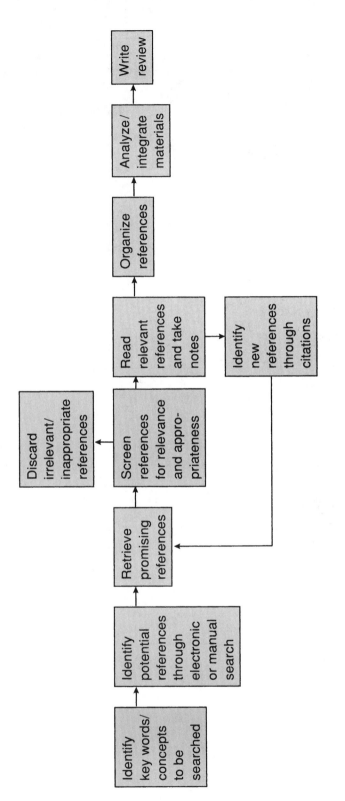

FIGURE 6-2. Flow of tasks in preparing a written research review

Copyright © 2001 by Lippincott Williams and Wilkins.
Instructor's Resource Manual and Testbank to Accompany Essentials of Nursing Research, fifth edition
by Denise F. Polit, Cheryl Tatano Beck and Bernadette P. Hungler.

TABLE 6-1. Examples of Stylistic Difficulties for Research Reviews

INAPPROPRIATE STYLE OR WORDING	RECOMMENDED CHANGE*
1. It is known that unmet expectations engender anxiety.	1. Several experts (Abraham, 1999; Lawrence, 2000) have asserted that unmet expectations engender anxiety
2. The woman who does not participate in childbirth preparation classes tends to manifest high degree of stress during labor.	2. Previous studies indicate that women who participate in preparation for childbirth classes manifest less stress during labor than those who do not (Klotz, 2000; McTygue, 1998).
3. Studies have proved that doctors and nurses do not fully understand the psychobiologic dynamics of recovery from a myocardial infarction.	3. The studies by Singleton (1999) and Fortune (2000) suggest that doctors and nurses do not fully understand the psychobiologic dynamics of recovery from a myocardial infarction.
4. Attitudes cannot be changed overnight.	4. Attitudes have been found to be relatively enduring attributes that cannot be changed overnight (O'Connell, 1999; Valentine, 2000).
5. Responsibility is an intrinsic stressor.	5. According to Doctor A. Cassard, an authority on stress, responsibility is an intrinsic stressor (Cassard, 1998, 1999).

*All references are fictitious.

Copyright © 2001 by Lippincott Williams and Wilkins.
Instructor's Resource Manual and Testbank to Accompany Essentials of Nursing Research, fifth edition
by Denise F. Polit, Cheryl Tatano Beck and Bernadette P. Hungler.

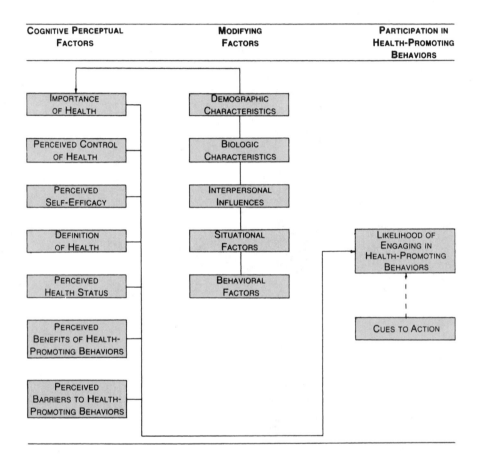

| COGNITIVE PERCEPTUAL FACTORS | MODIFYING FACTORS | PARTICIPATION IN HEALTH-PROMOTING BEHAVIORS |

IMPORTANCE OF HEALTH

PERCEIVED CONTROL OF HEALTH

PERCEIVED SELF-EFFICACY

DEFINITION OF HEALTH

PERCEIVED HEALTH STATUS

PERCEIVED BENEFITS OF HEALTH-PROMOTING BEHAVIORS

PERCEIVED BARRIERS TO HEALTH-PROMOTING BEHAVIORS

DEMOGRAPHIC CHARACTERISTICS

BIOLOGIC CHARACTERISTICS

INTERPERSONAL INFLUENCES

SITUATIONAL FACTORS

BEHAVIORAL FACTORS

LIKELIHOOD OF ENGAGING IN HEALTH-PROMOTING BEHAVIORS

CUES TO ACTION

FIGURE 7–1. The health promotion model (From Pender et al., 1990)

Copyright © 2001 by Lippincott Williams and Wilkins.
Instructor's Resource Manual and Testbank to Accompany Essentials of Nursing Research, fifth edition by Denise F. Polit, Cheryl Tatano Beck and Bernadette P. Hungler.

TABLE 7-1. Examples of Studies Linked to Conceptual Models of Nursing

CONCEPTUAL MODEL	RESEARCH QUESTION
King's Open System Model	What is the effect of a nurse–client transactional intervention on female adolescents' oral contraceptive adherence? (Hanna, 1993)
Levine's Conservation Model	What are the dimensions of fatigue as experienced by patients with congestive heart failure? (Schaefer & Potylycki, 1993)
Neuman's Health Care Systems Model	What is the relationship between mood symptoms and daytime ambulatory blood pressure during a 12-hour period in black female caregivers and noncaregivers? (Picot, Zauszniewski, Debanne, & Holston, 1999)
Orem's Model of Self-Care	What is the relationship between self-care agency and abuse on the one hand and physical and emotional health on the other among women in intimate relationships? (Campbell & Soeken, 1999)
Parse's Theory of Human Becoming	What are the factors that influence young women's perceptions of risk for sexually transmitted diseases? (Hutchinson, 1999)
Peplau's Interpersonal Relations Model	What are the factors influencing movement of nurse–patient dyads from Peplau's orientation phase to the working phase of the nurse–client relationship in a psychiatric setting? (Forchuk, Westwell, Martin, Azzapardi, Kosterewa-Tolman, & Hux, 1998)
Rogers' Science of Unitary Human Beings	What is the efficacy of a Rogerian-based intervention of therapeutic touch on anxiety, pain, and plasma T-lymphocyte concentration in burn patients? (Turner, Clark, Gauthier, & Williams, 1998)
Roy's Adaptation Model	Do formal cancer support groups help women to adapt to the physiological and psychosocial sequelae of breast cancer? (Samarel, Fawcett, Krippendorf, Piacentino, Eliasof, Hughes, Kowitski, & Siegler, 1998)

Copyright © 2001 by Lippincott Williams and Wilkins.
Instructor's Resource Manual and Testbank to Accompany Essentials of Nursing Research, fifth edition
by Denise F. Polit, Cheryl Tatano Beck and Bernadette P. Hungler.

TABLE 8-1. Dimensions of Quantitative Research Designs

DIMENSION	DESIGN	MAJOR FEATURES
Control over independent variable	Experimental	Manipulation of independent variable, control group, randomization
	Quasi-experimental	Manipulation of independent variable but no randomization or no control group
	Nonexperimental	No manipulation of independent variable
Type of group comparisons	Between-subjects	Participants in groups being compared are different people.
	Within-subjects	Participants in groups being compared are the same people.
Number of data collection points	Cross-sectional	Data collected at one point in time
	Longitudinal	Data collected at multiple points in time over extended period
Occurrence of independent and dependent variable	Retrospective	Study begins with dependent variable and looks backward for cause or influence.
	Prospective	Study begins with independent variable and looks forward for the effect.
Setting	Naturalistic	Data collected in a real-world setting
	Laboratory	Data collected in artificial, contrived setting

Copyright © 2001 by Lippincott Williams and Wilkins.
Instructor's Resource Manual and Testbank to Accompany Essentials of Nursing Research, fifth edition
by Denise F. Polit, Cheryl Tatano Beck and Bernadette P. Hungler.

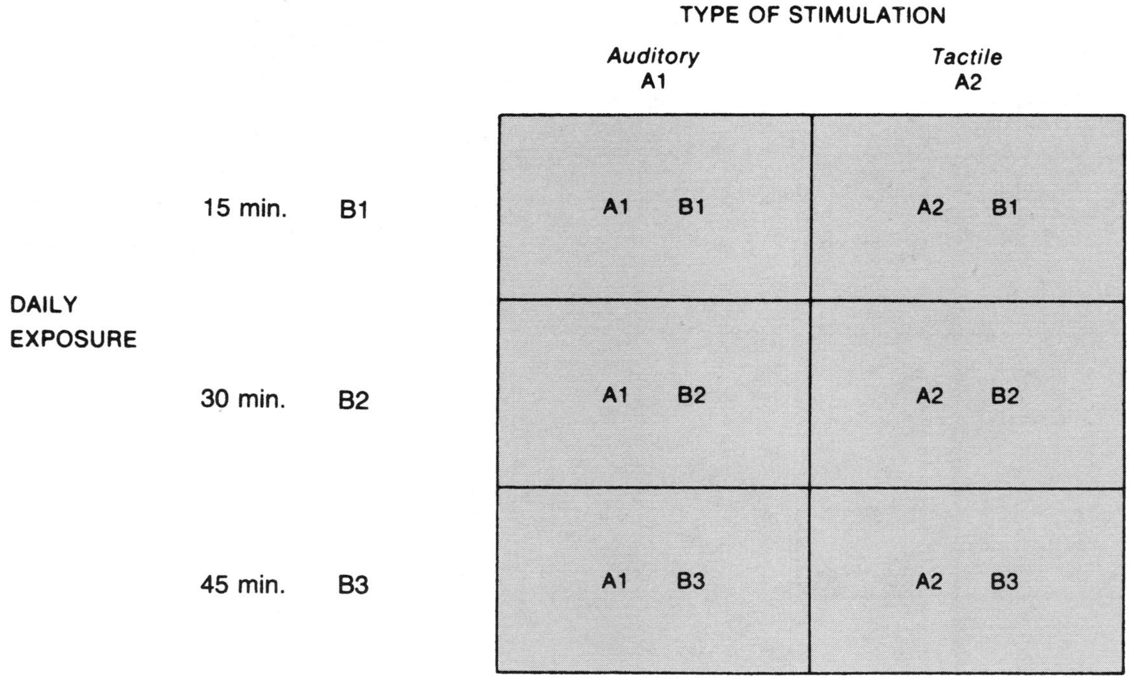

FIGURE 8-1. Schematic diagram of a factorial experiment

Copyright © 2001 by Lippincott Williams and Wilkins.
Instructor's Resource Manual and Testbank to Accompany Essentials of Nursing Research, fifth edition by Denise F. Polit, Cheryl Tatano Beck and Bernadette P. Hungler.

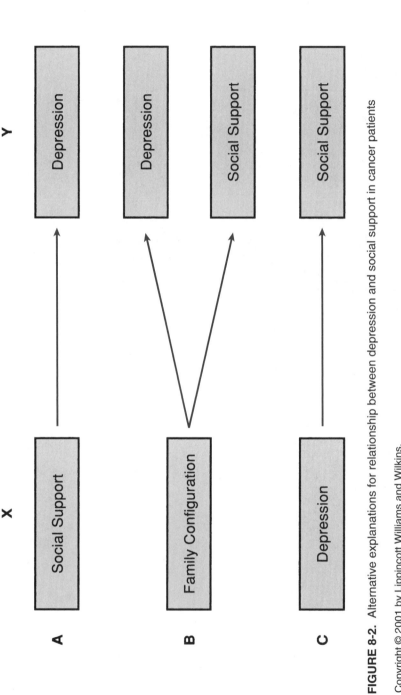

FIGURE 8-2. Alternative explanations for relationship between depression and social support in cancer patients

Copyright © 2001 by Lippincott Williams and Wilkins.
Instructor's Resource Manual and Testbank to Accompany Essentials of Nursing Research, fifth edition
by Denise F. Polit, Cheryl Tatano Beck and Bernadette P. Hungler.

TABLE 9-1. Overview of Qualitative Research Traditions

DISCIPLINE	DOMAIN	RESEARCH TRADITION	AREA OF INQUIRY
Anthropology	Culture	Ethnography	Holistic view of a culture
		Ethnoscience (cognitive anthropology)	Mapping of the cognitive world of a culture; a culture's shared meanings, semantic rules
Psychology or philosophy	Lived experience	Phenomenology	Experiences of individuals within their lifeworld
		Hermeneutics	Interpretations and meanings of individuals' experiences
Psychology	Behavior and events	Ethology	Behavior observed over time in natural context
		Ecological psychology	Behavior as influenced by the environment
Sociology	Social settings	Grounded theory	Social structural processes within a social setting
		Ethnomethodology	Manner by which shared agreement is achieved in social settings
Sociolinguistics	Human communication	Discourse analysis	Forms and rules of conversation

Copyright © 2001 by Lippincott Williams and Wilkins.
Instructor's Resource Manual and Testbank to Accompany Essentials of Nursing Research, fifth edition
by Denise F. Polit, Cheryl Tatano Beck and Bernadette P. Hungler.

TABLE 10-1. Numbers and Percentages of Students in Strata of a Population, Convenience Sample, and Quota Sample

	FRESHMEN	SOPHOMORES	JUNIORS	SENIORS	TOTAL
POPULATION					
Males	25 (2.5%)	25 (2.5%)	25 (2.5%)	25 (2.5%)	100 (10%)
Females	225 (22.5%)	225 (22.5%)	225 (22.5%)	225 (22.5%)	900 (90%)
TOTAL	250 (25%)	250 (25%)	250 (25%)	250 (25%)	1000 (100%)
CONVENIENCE SAMPLE					
Males	2 (1%)	4 (2%)	3 (1.5%)	1 (0.5%)	10 (5%)
Females	98 (49%)	36 (18%)	37 (18.5%)	19 (9.5%)	190 (95%)
TOTAL	100 (50%)	40 (20%)	40 (20%)	20 (10%)	200 (100%)
QUOTA SAMPLE					
Males	5 (2.5%)	5 (2.5%)	5 (2.5%)	5 (2.5%)	20 (10%)
Females	45 (22.5%)	45 (22.5%)	45 (22.5%)	45 (22.5%)	180 (90%)
TOTAL	50 (25%)	50 (25%)	50 (25%)	50 (25%)	200 (100%)

Copyright © 2001 by Lippincott Williams and Wilkins.
Instructor's Resource Manual and Testbank to Accompany Essentials of Nursing Research, fifth edition by Denise F. Polit, Cheryl Tatano Beck and Bernadette P. Hungler.

BOX 11-1 □ **EXAMPLES OF QUESTION TYPES**

Open-ended

- What led to your decision to stop smoking?
- What did you do when you discovered you had AIDS?

Closed-Ended

1. Dichotomous Question

Have you ever been hospitalized?

- ❏ 1. Yes
- ❏ 2. No

2. Multiple-Choice Question

How important is it to you to avoid a pregnancy at this time?

- ❏ 1. Extremely important
- ❏ 2. Very important
- ❏ 3. Somewhat important
- ❏ 4. Not at all important

3. "Cafeteria" Question

People have different opinions about the use of estrogen-replacement therapy for women in menopause. Which of the following statements best represents your point of view?

- ❏ 1. Estrogen replacement is dangerous and should be totally banned.
- ❏ 2. Estrogen replacement may have some undesirable side effects that suggests the need for caution in its use.
- ❏ 3. I am undecided about my views on estrogen-replacement therapy.
- ❏ 4. Estrogen replacement has many beneficial effects that merit its promotion.
- ❏ 5. Estrogen replacement is a wonder cure that should be administered routinely to menopausal women.

4. Rank-Order Question

People value different things about life. Below is a list of principles or ideals that are often cited when people are asked to name things they value most. Please indicate the order of importance of these values to you by placing a 1 beside the most important, 2 beside the next most important, and so forth.

- ❏ Achievement and success
- ❏ Family relationships
- ❏ Friendships and social interaction
- ❏ Health
- ❏ Money
- ❏ Religion

(continued)

Copyright © 2001 by Lippincott Williams and Wilkins.
Instructor's Resource Manual and Testbank to Accompany Essentials of Nursing Research, fifth edition by Denise F. Polit, Cheryl Tatano Beck and Bernadette P. Hungler.

BOX 11-1 ▢   *(Continued)*

5. Forced-Choice Question

Which statement most closely represents your point of view?

❏ 1. What happens to me is my own doing.
❏ 2. Sometimes I feel I don't have enough control over my life.

6. Rating Question

On a scale from 0 to 10, where 0 means extremely dissatisfied and 10 means extremely satisfied, how satisfied are you with the nursing care you received during your hospitalization?

Extremely dissatisfied   Extremely satisfied

            0 1 2 3 4 5 6 7 8 9 10

Copyright © 2001 by Lippincott Williams and Wilkins.

Instructor's Resource Manual and Testbank to Accompany Essentials of Nursing Research, fifth edition by Denise F. Polit, Cheryl Tatano Beck and Bernadette P. Hungler.

NURSE PRACTITIONERS

	7*	6	5	4	3	2	1	
competent								incompetent
worthless	1	2	3	4	5	6	7	valuable
important								unimportant
pleasant								unpleasant
bad								good
cold								warm
responsible								irresponsible
successful								unsuccessful

*The score values would not be printed on the form administered to actual subjects. The numbers are presented here solely for the purpose of illustrating how semantic differentials are scored.

FIGURE 11-1. Example of a semantic differential

Copyright © 2001 by Lippincott Williams and Wilkins.
Instructor's Resource Manual and Testbank to Accompany Essentials of Nursing Research, fifth edition by Denise F. Polit, Cheryl Tatano Beck and Bernadette P. Hungler.

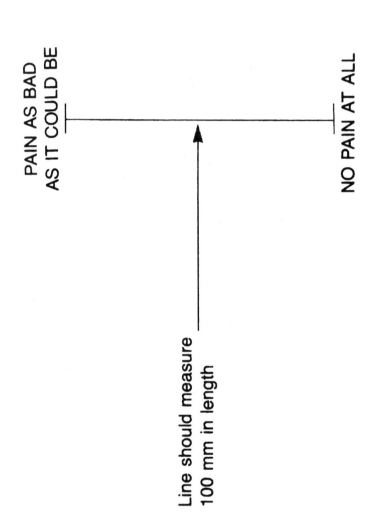

FIGURE 11-2. Example of a visual analog scale

Copyright © 2001 by Lippincott Williams and Wilkins.
Instructor's Resource Manual and Testbank to Accompany Essentials of Nursing Research, fifth edition
by Denise F. Polit, Cheryl Tatano Beck and Bernadette P. Hungler.

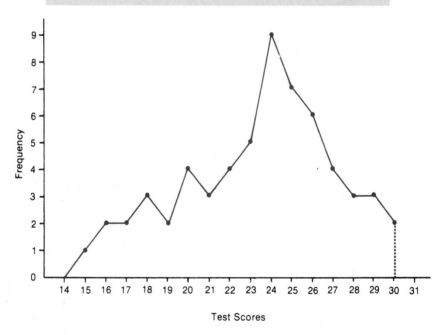

TABLE 13-2. Frequency Distribution of AIDS Knowledge Test Scores

SCORE	FREQUENCY	PERCENTAGE
15	1	1.7
16	2	3.3
17	2	3.3
18	3	5.0
19	2	3.3
20	4	6.7
21	3	5.0
22	4	6.7
23	5	8.3
24	9	15.0
25	7	11.7
26	6	10.0
27	4	6.7
28	3	5.0
29	3	5.0
30	2	3.3
	$N = 60$	100.0

FIGURE 13–1. Frequency polygon of AIDS knowledge test scores.

Copyright © 2001 by Lippincott Williams and Wilkins.
Instructor's Resource Manual and Testbank to Accompany Essentials of Nursing Research, fifth edition by Denise F. Polit, Cheryl Tatano Beck and Bernadette P. Hungler.

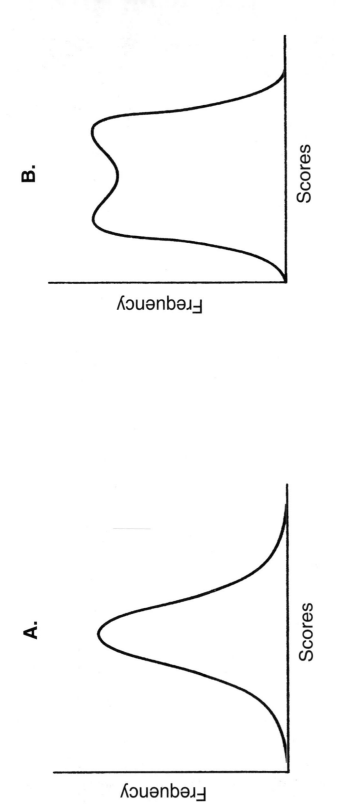

FIGURE 13-2. Example of symmetric distributions

Copyright © 2001 by Lippincott Williams and Wilkins.
Instructor's Resource Manual and Testbank to Accompany Essentials of Nursing Research, fifth edition
by Denise F. Polit, Cheryl Tatano Beck and Bernadette P. Hungler.

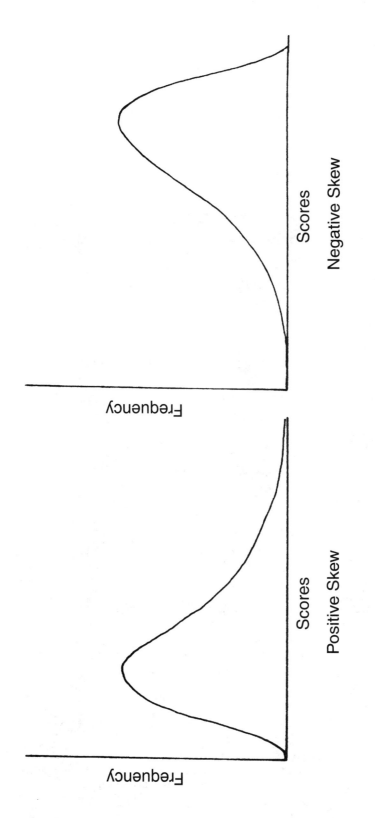

FIGURE 13-3. Examples of skewed distributions

Copyright © 2001 by Lippincott Williams and Wilkins.
Instructor's Resource Manual and Testbank to Accompany Essentials of Nursing Research, fifth edition
by Denise F. Polit, Cheryl Tatano Beck and Bernadette P. Hungler.

TABLE 13-3.	Example of Table Showing Frequency Distribution Information: Sample Characteristics in Study of the Effect of Relaxation Therapy on Preterm Labor Outcomes	
CATEGORY	N = 107	PERCENTAGE
Race/ethnicity	White: 92	86.0
	Nonwhite: 15	14.0
Marital status	Married: 76	71.0
	Unmarried: 31	29.0
Income	$25,000 or less: 33	31.4
	>$25,000 to 55,000: 36	34.3
	>$55,000: 36	34.3
Parity	Nullipara: 43	40.2
	Primipara: 44	41.1
	Multipara: 20	18.7

Adapted from Janke, J. (1999). The effect of relaxation therapy on preterm labor outcomes. *Journal of Obstetric, Gynecologic, and Neonatal Nursing, 28,* 255–263, Table 1.

Copyright © 2001 by Lippincott Williams and Wilkins.
Instructor's Resource Manual and Testbank to Accompany Essentials of Nursing Research, fifth edition by Denise F. Polit, Cheryl Tatano Beck and Bernadette P. Hungler.

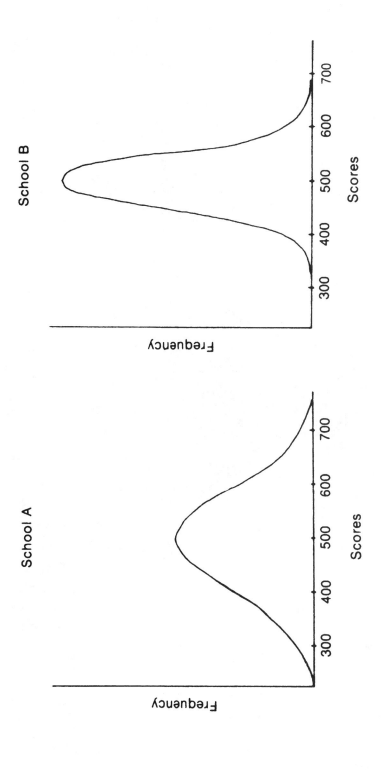

FIGURE 13-4. Two distributions of different variability

Copyright © 2001 by Lippincott Williams and Wilkins.
Instructor's Resource Manual and Testbank to Accompany Essentials of Nursing Research, fifth edition
by Denise F. Polit, Cheryl Tatano Beck and Bernadette P. Hungler.

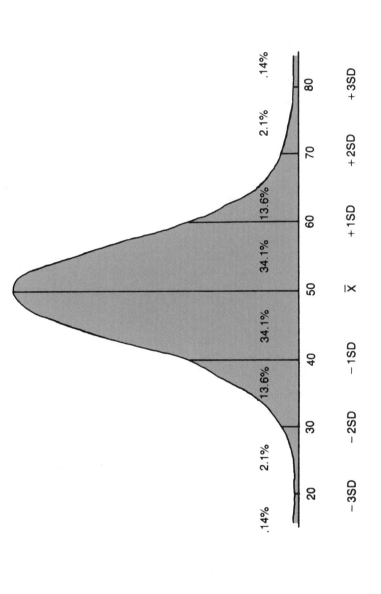

FIGURE 13-5. Standard deviations in a normal distribution

Copyright © 2001 by Lippincott Williams and Wilkins.
Instructor's Resource Manual and Testbank to Accompany Essentials of Nursing Research, fifth edition
by Denise F. Polit, Cheryl Tatano Beck and Bernadette P. Hungler.

TABLE 13-4. Example of Table Showing Central Tendency and Variability: Study of Mood and Blood Pressure Responses in Black Female Caregivers and Noncaregivers

CHARACTERISTICS	NONCAREGIVERS ($n = 38$) $\overline{X}$(SD)	CAREGIVERS ($n = 37$) $\overline{X}$(SD)
Anger	2.10 (1.38)	2.71 (1.45)
Anxiety	2.65 (1.66)	3.21 (1.57)
Sadness	3.53 (1.72)	3.96 (1.80)
Diastolic blood pressure	81.37 (9.32)	78.96 (10.63)
Systolic blood pressure	130.48 (14.24)	131.18 (17.51)

Adapted from Picot, S.F., Zauszniewski, J.A., Debanne, S.M., & Holston, E.C. (1999). Mood and blood pressure responses in black female caregivers and noncaregivers. *Nursing Research, 48,* 62–70, Table 2.

TABLE 13-5. Contingency Table for Gender and Smoking Status Relationship

SMOKING STATUS	GENDER Female N	Female %	Male N	Male %	Total N	Total %
Nonsmoker	₩₩ ₩₩ 10	45.4	₩₩ I 6	27.3	16	36.4
Light smoker	₩₩ III 8	36.4	₩₩ III 8	36.4	16	36.4
Heavy smoker	IIII 4	18.2	₩₩ III 8	36.4	12	27.3
TOTAL	22	50.0	22	50.0	44	100.0

Copyright © 2001 by Lippincott Williams and Wilkins.
Instructor's Resource Manual and Testbank to Accompany Essentials of Nursing Research, fifth edition by Denise F. Polit, Cheryl Tatano Beck and Bernadette P. Hungler.

TABLE 13-6. Example of a Contingency Table: Study of Dyspnea in Relation to Diagnoses and Dispositions

DIAGNOSIS	DYSPNEA		NO DYSPNEA		TOTAL n
	%	n	%	n	
COPD	78.2	187	21.8	52	239
Asthma	87.6	346	12.4	49	395
Mixed COPD and asthma	66.7	12	33.3	6	18
Restrictive	71.4	10	28.6	4	14
Congestive heart failure	61.6	197	38.4	123	320
TOTAL	76.3	752	23.7	234	986

COPD, chronic obstructive pulmonary disease.
Adapted from Parshall M.B. (1999). Adult emergency visits for chronic cardiorespiratory disease: Does dyspnea matter? *Nursing Research, 48,* 62–70, Table 2.

Copyright © 2001 by Lippincott Williams and Wilkins.
Instructor's Resource Manual and Testbank to Accompany Essentials of Nursing Research, fifth edition
by Denise F. Polit, Cheryl Tatano Beck and Bernadette P. Hungler.

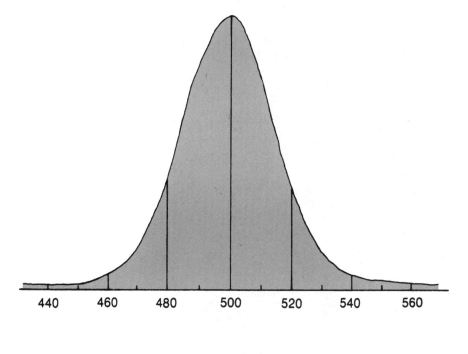

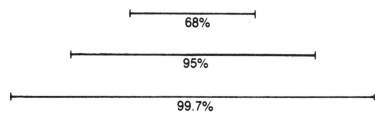

FIGURE 13-6. Sampling distribution of a mean

Copyright © 2001 by Lippincott Williams and Wilkins.
Instructor's Resource Manual and Testbank to Accompany Essentials of Nursing Research,
fifth edition by Denise F. Polit, Cheryl Tatano Beck and Bernadette P. Hungler.

The actual situation is that the null hypothesis is:

	True	False
The researcher calculates a test statistic and decides that the null hypothesis is: True (Null accepted)	Correct decision	Type II error
False (Null rejected)	Type I error	Correct decision

FIGURE 13-7. Outcomes of statistical decision making

Copyright © 2001 by Lippincott Williams and Wilkins.
Instructor's Resource Manual and Testbank to Accompany Essentials of Nursing Research, fifth edition by Denise F. Polit, Cheryl Tatano Beck and Bernadette P. Hungler.

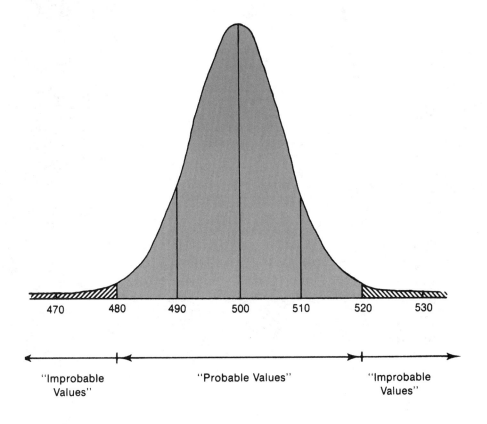

FIGURE 13-8. Sampling distribution for hypothesis testing example of SAT scores

Copyright © 2001 by Lippincott Williams and Wilkins.
Instructor's Resource Manual and Testbank to Accompany Essentials of Nursing Research, fifth edition by Denise F. Polit, Cheryl Tatano Beck and Bernadette P. Hungler.

TABLE 13-13. Guide to Widely Used Bivariate Statistical Tests

NAME	TEST STATISTIC	PURPOSE	MEASUREMENT LEVEL* IV	MEASUREMENT LEVEL* DV
PARAMETRIC TESTS				
t-test for independent groups	t	To test the difference between two independent group means	Nominal	Interval, ratio
t-test for dependent groups	t	To test the difference between two dependent group means	Nominal	Interval, ratio
Analysis of variance (ANOVA)	F	To test the difference among the means of three or more independent groups, or of more than one independent variable	Nominal	Interval, ratio
Repeated measures ANOVA	F	To test the difference among means of three or more related groups or sets of scores	Nominal	Interval, ratio
Pearson's r	r	To test the existence of a relationship between two variables	Interval, ratio	Interval, ratio
NONPARAMETRIC TESTS				
Chi-squared test	χ^2	To test the difference in proportions in two or more independent groups	Nominal	Nominal
Mann-Whitney U-test	U	To test the difference in ranks of scores on two independent groups	Nominal	Ordinal
Kruskal-Wallis test	H	To test the difference in ranks of scores of three or more independent groups	Nominal	Ordinal
Wilcoxon signed ranks test	T (Z)	To test the difference in ranks of scores of two related groups	Nominal	Ordinal
Friedman test	χ^2	To test the difference in ranks of scores of three or more related groups	Nominal	Ordinal
Phi coefficient	ϕ	To test the magnitude of a relationship between two dichotomous variables	Nominal	Nominal
Spearman's rank-order correlation	r_s	To test the existence of a relationship between two variables	Ordinal	Ordinal

*Measurement level of the independent variable (IV) and dependent variable (DV).

Copyright © 2001 by Lippincott Williams and Wilkins.
Instructor's Resource Manual and Testbank to Accompany Essentials of Nursing Research, fifth edition by Denise F. Polit, Cheryl Tatano Beck and Bernadette P. Hungler.

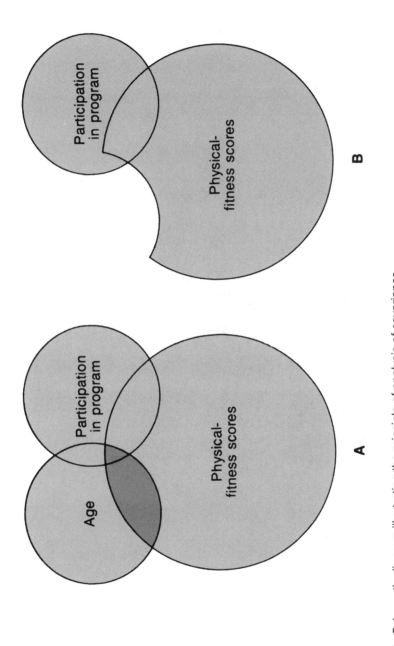

FIGURE 13-9. Schematic diagram illustrating the principle of analysis of covariance

Copyright © 2001 by Lippincott Williams and Wilkins.
Instructor's Resource Manual and Testbank to Accompany Essentials of Nursing Research, fifth edition
by Denise F. Polit, Cheryl Tatano Beck and Bernadette P. Hungler.

TABLE 13-14. Guide to Widely Used Multivariate Statistical Analyses

NAME	PURPOSE	MEASUREMENT LEVEL*			NUMBER OF:		
		IV	DV	COV	IVs	DVs	COVs
Multiple correlation, regression	To test the relationship between two or more IVs and 1 DV; to predict a DV from two or more IVs	N, I, R	I, R		2+	1	
Analysis of covariance (ANCOVA)	To test the difference between the means of two or more groups, while controlling for one or more covariate	N	I, R	N, I, R	1+	1	1+
Multivariate analysis of variance (MANOVA)	To test the difference between the means of two or more groups for two or more DVs simultaneously	N	I, R		1+	2+	
Multivariate analysis of covariance (MANCOVA)	To test the difference between the means of two or more groups for two or more DVs simultaneously, while controlling for one or more covariate	N	I, R	N, I, R	1+	2+	1+
Factor analysis	To determine the dimensionality or structure of a set of variables						
Discriminant analysis	To test the relationship between two or more IVs and one DV; to predict group membership; to classify cases into groups	N, I, R	N		2+	1	
Logistic regression	To test the relationship betweenDS two or more IVs and one DV; to predict the probability of an event; to estimate relative risk (odds ratios)	N, I, R	N		2+	1	

*Measurement level of the independent variable (IV), dependent variable (DV), and covariates (Cov): N = nominal, I = interval, R = ratio.

Copyright © 2001 by Lippincott Williams and Wilkins.
Instructor's Resource Manual and Testbank to Accompany Essentials of Nursing Research, fifth edition by Denise F. Polit, Cheryl Tatano Beck and Bernadette P. Hungler.

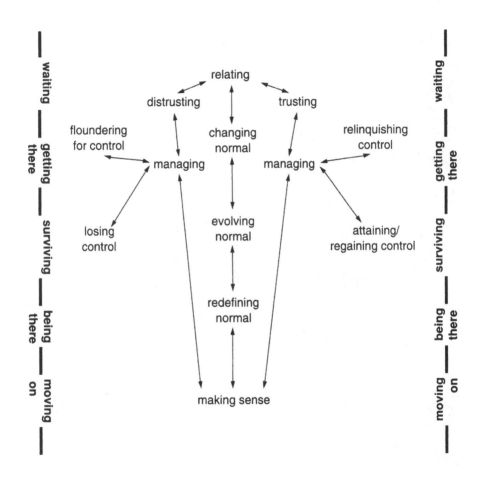

FIGURE 14-3. King and Jensen's (1994) model of preserving the self during cardiac surgery (reprinted with permission)

Copyright © 2001 by Lippincott Williams and Wilkins.
Instructor's Resource Manual and Testbank to Accompany Essentials of Nursing Research, fifth edition by Denise F. Polit, Cheryl Tatano Beck and Bernadette P. Hungler.

TABLE 16-2. Criteria for Comparative Evaluation Phase of the Stetler Model of Research Utilization*

1. Fit of setting
   Similarity of characteristics of sample to your client population
   Similarity of study's environment to the one in which you work
2. Feasibility
   Potential risks of implementation to patients, staff, and the organization
   Readiness for change among those who would be involved in a change in practice
   Resource requirements and availability
3. Current Practice
   Congruency of the study with your theoretical basis for current practice behavior
4. Substantiating Evidence
   Availability of confirming evidence from other studies
   Availability of confirming evidence from a meta-analysis or integrative review

---

*Adapted from Stetler, C. B. (1994). Refinement of the Stetler/Marram model for application of research findings to practice. *Nursing Outlook, 42*, 15–25.

Copyright © 2001 by Lippincott Williams and Wilkins.
Instructor's Resource Manual and Testbank to Accompany Essentials of Nursing Research, fifth edition by Denise F. Polit, Cheryl Tatano Beck and Bernadette P. Hungler.

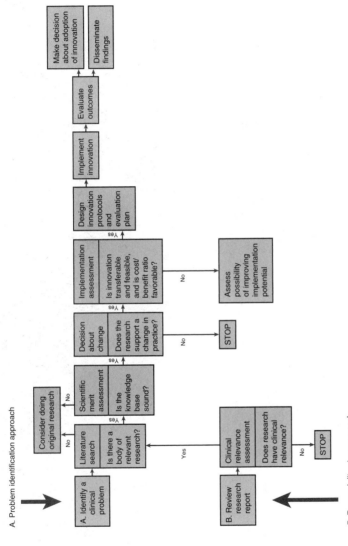

FIGURE 16-1. A model for research utilization

Copyright © 2001 by Lippincott Williams and Wilkins.
Instructor's Resource Manual and Testbank to Accompany Essentials of Nursing Research, fifth edition
by Denise F. Polit, Cheryl Tatano Beck and Bernadette P. Hungler.

Testbank Data CD Instructions

For use on IBM PC compatibles and Macintosh systems (with or without WIN-DOWS) equipped with a Super Drive

INTRODUCTION

This electronic test-generating program contains plain .RTF word-processing files for:

Instructor's Resource Manual and Testbank to Accompany Essentials of Nursing Research: Methods, Appraisal, and Utilization, Fifth Edition.

Test items for each chapter are stored in separate files and all ANSWERS appear together in ONE file. For example, test items for Chapter 7 can be found under the file name that would include the number "7" or "07". CD files can be used with any commercial word processing software. The files mirror the printed version (if applicable) with the exception that underlined (or italicized) material is roman and subscripts and superscripts may not ascend or descend. For example, CO_2 may appear as CO2. You will have to use your own word processor to make necessary adjustments. You may also use test items as is, or you may alter them in accordance with your own specifications.

HARDWARE AND SOFTWARE REQUIREMENTS

Word processing software for the IBM PC (or compatible) or Macintosh systems complete with memory and include hardware necessary to run any *type* of word processing software.

INSTRUCTIONS

Before using any of the files on the CD, make a copy of the master CD onto a new **formatted** *blank* disk or CD by opening your word processing program and copying files as you normally would. (You may have to copy files to your hard drive before making an additional disk copy, but a CD burner is required to make a duplicate CD.)

If your word processor has a **Text IN/OUT** feature, you should use this when loading files because they are stored in generic .RTF (DOS) text file format and would be much easier to use. Otherwise, retrieve them exactly the same as you would any other document on a CD.

1. To use actual Testbank files, start your word-processing software as you normally would and re-set your margins. You must use your own word processing software in order to be able to view or "edit" files.

2. Files may be stored with a hard return at the end of every line. If you plan to add, delete, or change text within a line, you will need to use your backspace key to delete any hard returns in the surrounding text or search and remove them. Your word-processing software can then wrap words from one line to another *automatically* based on your margin set-up.

3. When you have modified files, save them on your hard drive, a blank CD or **formatted** disk. For preservation, do *not* re-save any documents you've altered on the original Testbank CD.

Copyright © 2001 by Lippincott Williams & Wilkins. For technical assistance, please call Lippincott Williams & Wilkins Software Support at 1-800-348-0854 between 10:00 am. and 6:00 pm. EST. This item is for instructors to use in classes where they have adopted the accompanying text only. Such copies should show the copyright notice printed above and any sales for further distribution are strictly prohibited. IBM is a registered trademark of International Business Machines Corporation.